Diet Plan For I

Learn how to manage liver disease with this step-by-step guide. Follow the food plan and selected recipes to improve your overall health and well-being.

ASTRID MESKILL

© Copyright 2021 by ASTRID MESKILL- All rights reserved.

This document is geared towards providing exact and reliable information in regards to the topic and issue covered. The publication is sold with the idea that the publisher is not required to render accounting, officially permitted, or otherwise, qualified services. If advice is necessary, legal or professional, a practiced individual in the profession should be ordered.

- From a Declaration of Principles which was accepted and approved equally by a Committee of the American Bar Association and a Committee of Publishers and Associations.

In no way is it legal to reproduce, duplicate, or transmit any part of this document in either electronic means or in printed format. Recording of this publication is strictly prohibited, and any storage of this document is not allowed unless with written permission from the publisher. All rights reserved.

The information provided herein is stated to be truthful and consistent, in that any liability, in terms of inattention or otherwise, by any usage or abuse of any policies, processes, or Instructions contained within is the solitary and utter responsibility of the recipient reader. Under no circumstances will any legal responsibility or blame be held against the publisher for any reparation, damages, or monetary loss due to the information herein, either directly or indirectly.

Respective authors own all copyrights not held by the publisher.

The information herein is offered for informational purposes solely and is universal as such. The presentation of the information is without a contract or any type of guarantee assurance.

The trademarks that are used are without any consent, and the publication of the trademark is without permission or backing by the trademark owner. All trademarks and brands within this book are for clarifying purposes only and are owned by the owners themselves, not affiliated with this document.

Table of Content

Introduction 6

Chapter 1. Understanding the Concept of Diet 10

1.1 Importance Of A Balanced Diet 15

Chapter 2. What is Fatty Liver Disease? 17

2.1 Liver's Functions 17

2.2 Alcoholic Liver Disease 20

2.3 Alcoholic Fatty Liver Disease 21

2.4 Alcoholic Hepatitis 22

2.5 Cirrhosis 22

2.6 Non-Alcoholic Fatty Liver Disease 23

Chapter 3. Causes Of Fatty Liver 27

3.1 Causes Of Fatty Liver Disease 28

3.2 Signs And Symptoms 30

3.3 Diagnosis And Tests 32

Chapter 4. Problems Due To A Fatty Liver Disease 36

4.1 Internal (Variceal) Bleeding 37

4.2 Toxins Build-Up In The Brain (Encephalopathy) 38

4.3 Abdomen Fluid Accumulation (Ascites) Associated Kidney Failure 41

4.4 Liver Cancer 45

4.5 Increased Vulnerability To Infection 48

Chapter 5. Fatty Liver Disease Diet 49

5.1 Foods For A Fatty Liver 51

5.2 Foods To Avoid 64

Chapter 6. Recipes for Nourishing the Fatty Liver 70

6.1 Breakfast Recipes For Fatty Liver 71

6.2 Liver Friendly Appetizers, Soups and Salads..*89*

6.3 Lunch Recipes For Fatty Liver *145*

6.4 Fatty Liver Friendly Dinner Recipes..*162*

Conclusion **202**

Introduction

The liver's most remarkable feature is its ability to heal and recover from harm in ways that other organs, such as our heart & kidneys, cannot. If you're courageous enough to create and keep to lifestyle improvements and a healthy, whole foods diet, you can heal anything that ails you.

The fatty liver disorder is characterized by the presence of excess fat in the liver. It's possible that the doctor would refer to it as hepatic steatosis.

You're more likely to have it if you drink a lot. Too much alcohol causes fat to build up within the liver cells over time. This makes the liver's job more difficult.

Even if you don't consume a lot of alcohol, you might develop fatty liver disease.

In the care of nonalcoholic fatty liver disease, lifestyle changes, particularly nutritional guidelines, are important (NAFLD). Weight reduction and improvement in the clinical image of NAFLD can be achieved with a well-balanced, restrictive diet adapted to individual needs. Low-calorie diets abundant in unsaturated fatty acids & natural antioxidants are suggested (vitamins A and C). Carbohydrates can account for 40–50% of overall dietary energy, according to nutritional guidelines for patients with NAFLD. It's a good idea to eat more complex carbohydrates that are high in dietary fiber. Excessive fructose intake induced by high nonalcoholic beverage consumption among subjects in developing countries plays a significant role in NAFLD's etiology. Fructose use stimulates de novo lipogenesis, which leads to the formation of fatty liver. Easy carbohydrates do not account for more than 10% of overall energy consumption.

Steatosis, hepatocellular ballooning, the development of apoptosis/necrosis, Mallory bodies and inflammation are histological characteristics of nonalcoholic fatty-liver disease (NAFLD). Nonalcoholic steatohepatitis (NASH) affects 10–20 percent of patients with NAFLD and can progress to cirrhosis & hepatocellular carcinoma. Since obesity, insulin resistance, hypertension, or dyslipidemia are all symptoms of the metabolic syndrome, NAFLD is often followed by obesity, hypertension, insulin resistance or dyslipidemia. As a result, dietary control and therapeutic activity are critical components of NAFLD treatment.

Because of its elevated incidence, nonalcoholic fatty liver disease (NAFLD) seems to be a significant public health issue. Obesity, type 2 diabetes mellitus (DM2), hypertension, hyperlipidemia, insulin resistance, and metabolic syndrome are also linked to nonalcoholic fatty liver disease. Nonalcoholic fatty liver disease (NAFLD) encompasses a wide clinical range spanning from steatosis to steatohepatitis (NASH), including various degrees of liver fibrosis, cirrhosis, and hepatocellular carcinoma in between (HCC). While there is no strong agreement on NAFLD's pharmacotherapy at this point, it is clear that clinical interventions should emphasize behavioral improvements. Diet and exercise programs are also the first lines of treatment, and trials have demonstrated that a balanced diet and weight reduction can be enough to slow disease development in NAFLD's early phases. Despite strong evidence that dietary changes are successful, the diet's scope and structure have yet to be determined.

Furthermore, patients often refuse to adhere to food recommendations. As a result, straightforward, multidisciplinary dietary recommendations that target disease mechanisms are needed. Furthermore, recent studies are gradually encouraging a customized diet strategy and the role of artificial intelligence (AI) in this. This thesis's focus was to look into the function of nutrients in NAFLD's pathophysiology, with a concentration on diet design.

Chapter 1. Understanding the Concept of Diet

A particular diet to which an individual complies to lose weight or for medical purposes.

Diet was first used in English in the thirteenth century. Its initial definition was "habitually taken food & drink," as in modern English. However, the diet was often used to indicate the "way of life" in the Middle & Early Modern English times. Diet's Greek ancestor diaita is derived from the term diaitasthan, which means "to lead one's life," originally meant "to lead one's life." Diaita has also been a more precise word in Greek for a way of life recommended by a physician, some regimen or a diet.

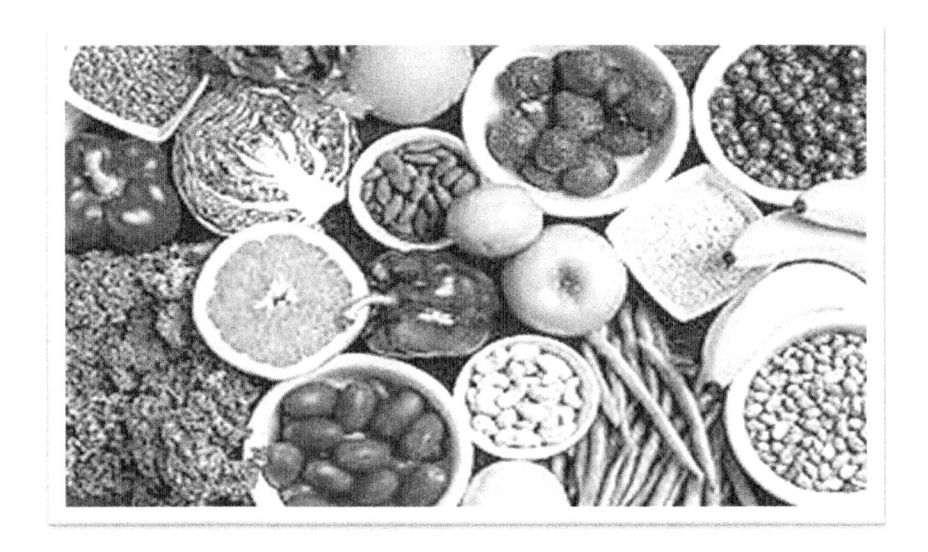

Diet is a concept tossed around so often that most people are unaware of what it entails. Diet may be seen as a negative concept, but this should not be the case. Diet can be related to a person's actual food consumption rather than relying exclusively on restraint or "going on a diet."

The phrase "diet" conjures up images of constraints in most people's minds. When you're on a diet, you're excluding or reducing those ingredients from your everyday routine.

Does the term "diet" conjure up images of a hectic weight-loss plan?

If something happens to you, you're not lonely. Remember the usage of the word "diet" in the advertisement of nutritional products—it typically applies to low-calorie diets like diet soda.

This title, however, has another sense. Diet may also apply to the food and drink an individual eats regularly and the mental and physical problems that follow eating. Nutrition entails more than only consuming a "healthy" diet; it often entails nourishment in all levels. It includes our experiences with our relatives, mates, nature (the environment), individual bodies, cultures, and the rest of the world.

Diet is better described as the food that an individual

absorbs regularly. It's smart to think about a diet as a noun rather than a verb while attempting to describe it. These factors make up a person's food, whether they make positive or poor decisions. The ultimate aim is to enable individuals to make the healthiest decisions available to enhance their overall well-being.

Unique diets that exist today include:

- Vegetarian
- Ketogenic
- Vegan
- Gluten-Free
- Blood Type Diet
- Paleo
- Mediterranean

Each one includes foods that are eaten on a daily basis. There may be several variations, but the diet is based on a number of staple foods.

A clear example is a Mediterranean diet. Unique items such as olive oil, almonds, seeds, seafood, whole wheat, spices, and some plants may be used in this diet.

The Mediterranean diet is a clear definition of a well-balanced, healthy diet.

A diet like this promotes better fitness, increased vitality, and increased energy. It is also popular for reducing cholesterol and helps to fight a variety of infections and health problems. It also tends to avoid heart failure, type 2 diabetes, and cognitive loss.

Processed and manufactured foods, on the other hand, can make up a person's diet. They can consume a significant amount of fast food and processed goods. These are poor decisions because they are the polar opposite of a balanced lifestyle. Obesity, cardiac disease, diabetes, and a number of other health issues may arise from this action.

How Does Diet Planning Works?

Diets are often based on short weight loss and fat loss. On the other hand, a diet schedule is personalized to a person's health condition, weight, and lifestyle, as well as their weight loss & health objectives.

For a healthier lifestyle, the value of a well-balanced diet cannot be overstated. Maintaining a proper diet and taking into account all of the necessary nutrients needed by the body will lead to a healthier lifestyle. A good meal schedule will help you reach your target body weight and lower your risk of chronic diseases, including diabetes, heart disease, and cancer.

What does it mean to eat a well-balanced diet?

But, precisely, what is a well-balanced diet? Simply put, it's a diet that provides the nutrients necessary for your body to work properly. Diet is essential since it ensures that the correct number of calories are consumed. When you eat a large range of calorie-dense foods like new vegetables and fruits, whole grains, and proteins, the body gets the nutrients it needs.

Calories

Calories are a calculation of a food's energy value. Calories are burnt as you walk, dream, or breathe after you consume something. A person's body weight maintenance may necessitate about 2000 calories per day on average. In general, a person's calorie intake is influenced by their gender, age, and level of physical activity. Males, on the other hand, need more calories than females. People who exercise regularly need more calories than someone who does not. It's also vital to bear in mind that the origins of calories are just as significant as the amount. Completing your diet with wasted calories, or calories that have little nutritious meaning, would not benefit you either way. Foods that are high in empty calories include:

- Sugar
- Cookies
- Pizza
- Butter
- Cakes
- Ice cream
- Energy drinks

1.1 Importance Of A Balanced Diet

Feeling better, getting more stamina, enhancing your fitness, and raising your morale benefit from eating a balanced diet. A person's general well-being and well-being depends on a good diet, physical exercise, and balanced body weight.

There's no denying the significance of eating nutritious foods in your existence. You may be susceptible to illnesses, illness, or even fatigue if you do not maintain a good diet for a safe body. The value of healthy food for infants, in particular, must be emphasized since they might otherwise be vulnerable to a variety of growth and developmental issues. Heart disease, asthma, stroke, and diabetes are three of the more prominent health conditions induced by a lack of a well-balanced diet.

Physical activity helps treat various wellness issues and promotes emotional health by lowering fatigue, depression, and discomfort. Metabolic syndrome, stroke, elevated blood pressure, arthritis, and anxiety will all be prevented with regular exercise.

Chapter 2. What is Fatty Liver Disease?

Fatty liver disease (FLD), commonly named hepatic steatosis, is a syndrome in which the liver builds up extra fat. There are also little or minimal signs.

There can be tiredness or inflammation in the upper side of the abdomen on occasion. Cirrhosis, liver disease, and esophageal varices are also possible complications.

2.1 Liver's Functions

The liver is an important organ that serves a set of life-sustaining roles. • The liver secretes bile, which supports digestion.

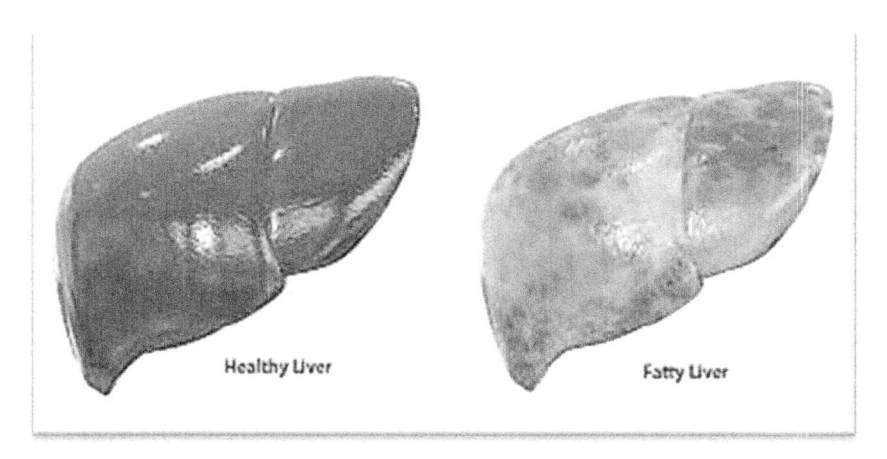

- Produces proteins for the human body.
- Iron is contained in this piece.
- It turns food into energy.

- Produces substances that aid in blood clotting (stick to heal wounds).
- Makes immunity factors and removes bacteria and chemicals (substances that can damage the body) from the blood, which helps you avoid infections.

What is fatty liver disease?

Steatosis (fatty liver disease) is a common disorder triggered by an accumulation of fat in the liver. There is a substantial proportion of fat in a balanced liver. When fat accounts for 5% – 10% of your liver's weight, it becomes a challenge.

What causes fatty liver disorder so dangerous?

Fatty liver disorder seldom causes serious complications or impairs the liver's ability to act normally. Fatty liver disorder worsens with time for 7 percent to 30% of those who develop it. It is divided into three stages:

1. The liver gets inflamed (swollen), causing tissue harm. Steatohepatitis is the name for this point.
2. When the liver is harmed, scar tissue develops. Fibrosis is the medical name for this disease.
3. Scar tissue replaces healthy tissue in significant numbers. Cirrhosis of the liver is evident at this point.

Cirrhosis of the liver is a disease that affects the liver.

Cirrhosis of the liver is caused by serious liver injury. The liver's activity is slowed by the strong scar tissue that covers healthy liver tissue. It has the ability to totally shut down liver activity. Cirrhosis may result in liver cancer and liver failure.

Hepatic steatosis is another term for fatty liver. It develops as the liver gets clogged with fat. Tiny quantities of fat in the liver are common, but too many may be detrimental to your wellbeing.

The liver is the body's second-largest organ. It assists in the absorption of nutrients from food and alcohol and the elimination of toxic compounds from the bloodstream.

Too much fat in the liver will lead to inflammation, which can weaken and mark your liver. This scarring will contribute to liver failure in serious cases.

The non-alcoholic fatty liver syndrome affects those who do not use a ton of alcohol (NAFLD). According to investigators in the World Journal of Gastroenterology, NAFLD impacts up to 25% to 30% of the United States and European population.

Forms Of Fatty Liver Disease

There are two main forms of fatty liver disease:

2.2 Alcoholic Liver Disease

Alcoholic fatty liver syndrome develops as a fatty liver forms in someone who takes a lot of alcohol (AFLD). The buildup of fat in the liver due to excessive drinking is referred to as alcoholic fatty liver. (One glass a day for women and two to three drinks a day for men is called light drinking.) This form of liver disorder affects approximately 5% of citizens in the United States.

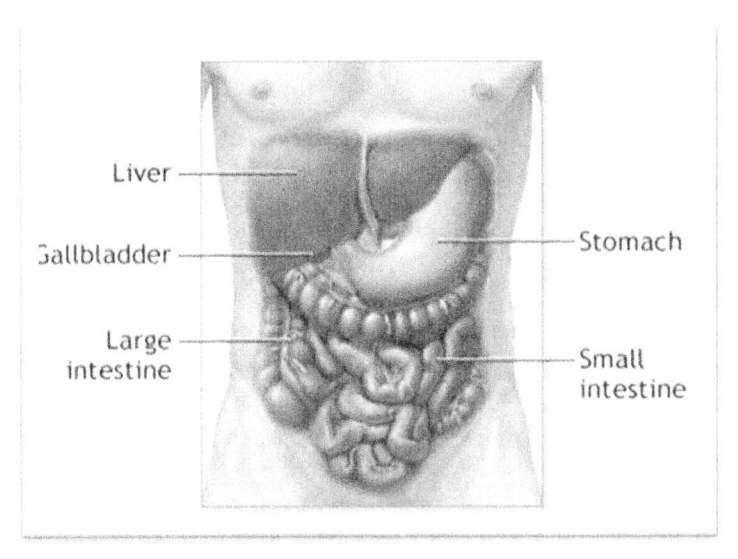

Fatty liver, alcoholic hepatitis, and cirrhosis are the three forms of liver disorder attributed to alcohol use. The fatty liver disorder progresses following a spell with excessive drinking that is normally reversible with abstinence. If abstinence or moderation is preserved, fatty liver is not thought to predispose a person to any permanent liver disease type. Alcoholic hepatitis is a serious cause of alcohol-induced liver damage that happens after a high amount of alcohol is consumed over a lengthy period of time. The seriousness of alcoholic hepatitis will vary from asymptomatic biochemical changes to liver disease and death. Cirrhosis is distinguished by substituting the usual hepatic parenchyma with dense bands of fibrous tissue with regenerative nodules, culminating in liver failure and portal hypertension.

Stages of ARLD

ARLD is categorized into three levels, but there is always overlap between them. These steps are described in detail below.

2.3 Alcoholic Fatty Liver Disease

And though it's just for a few days, drinking a lot of alcohol will cause fat to build up in the liver.

This is the first step of ARLD which is known as an alcoholic fatty liver disorder.

The fatty liver disorder has few signs, but it's a significant indication if you're consuming too much alcohol.

The fatty liver disorder should be treated. If you don't drink for two weeks, your liver could be back to usual.

2.4 Alcoholic Hepatitis

Alcoholic hepatitis, which is not the same as viral hepatitis, is a possibly lethal disease induced by long-term alcohol consumption.

When this happens, it may be the first time individuals realize they're harming their liver with alcohol.

Alcoholic hepatitis is a less prevalent complication of consuming a significant alcohol volume in a brief span of time.

Mild alcoholic hepatitis induces liver harm that is typically reversible once you stop drinking for good.

Severe alcoholic hepatitis, on the other hand, is a life-threatening condition.

Many people in the UK suffer from the disease each year, although certain people are only diagnosed with liver failure after their condition has advanced to this stage.

2.5 Cirrhosis

Cirrhosis is a level of ARLD in which the liver is deeply scarred. There might be no apparent signs even at this point.

While it's not always reversible, abstaining from alcohol will help you live longer by preventing more injury and extending the life expectancy.

An individual with cirrhosis induced by alcohol that does not quit drinking has a somewhat under 50% probability of surviving for another 5 years.

2.6 Non-Alcoholic Fatty Liver Disease

The non-alcoholic fatty liver disorder impacts those who may not consume excessively. In the United States, one in every three people and one in every ten adolescents have the disease. The precise origin of non-alcoholic liver disease is yet to be discovered. Obesity and diabetes are two conditions that will raise the risk.

Non-alcoholic fatty liver disease is a catch-all word for many liver disorders that impact people who don't consume alcohol. NAFLD is distinguished by an abundance of fat accumulated in liver cells, as the name suggests.

NAFLD is becoming more popular across the world, especially in Western countries. It is the most prevalent type of chronic liver disease in the United States, impacting roughly one-quarter of the country.

Non-alcoholic steatohepatitis (NASH) is an aggressive type of fatty liver disease characterized by liver inflammation that may lead to advanced scarring and liver failure in certain people with NAFLD. This harm is close to that created by excessive alcohol intake.

Non-alcoholic fatty liver disease is a very serious illness that applies to a category of disorders under which individuals who consume little or little alcohol develop extra fat in their liver. The most prevalent type of NAFLD is fatty liver, which is a non-serious disease. Fat accumulates of the liver cells in the fatty liver. While possessing fat in the liver seems rare, it is unlikely to affect its own liver. Non-alcoholic steatohepatitis is a dangerous disease that affects a limited percentage of individuals with NAFLD (NASH). Fat deposition is linked to liver cell inflammation and varying degrees of scarring in NASH. NASH is a possibly fatal disease that causes extensive scarring and cirrhosis of the liver. Cirrhosis happens when the liver is seriously injured, and the liver cells are eventually replaced by scar tissue, stopping the liver from working properly. Cirrhosis patients will undergo a liver transplant in the future.

NAFLD stands for non-alcoholic fatty liver disease, which applies to a category of diseases triggered by a buildup of fat in liver. It is more prevalent in overweight or obese individuals.

Fat should be minimal in a balanced liver. Up to one of every three individuals in the UK is thought to have NAFLD, which is characterized by tiny concentrations of fat in the liver.

Early-stage NAFLD is normally harmless, although as it progresses, it may inflict significant liver damage, including cirrhosis.

High amounts of fat in the liver are related to a greater incidence of major health conditions, including asthma, high blood pressure, and kidney failure.

NAFLD raises the chances of having cardiac attacks if you do have diabetes.

It is important to prevent NAFLD from worsening and reduce fat in the liver if it is diagnosed and treated early on.

Non-Alcoholic Fatty Liver Disease Stages

NAFLD progresses through four phases.

The majority of people would only develop the first level,

which they would typically be ignorant of.

If not identified and treated, it will develop and potentially contribute to liver injury in a limited amount of instances.

Simple Fatty Liver (Steatosis) – a comparatively harmless fat buildup in the liver cells which can only be identified during experiments conducted for another cause

Non-Alcoholic Steatohepatitis (NASH) – a more severe type of NAFLD in which the liver has been inflamed; it is reported that up to 5% of the UK population suffers from this disease.

Fibrosis – Scar tissue forms around the liver and surrounding blood vessels due to chronic inflammation, but the liver continues to work normally.

Cirrhosis – The most serious stage occurs after years of infection, where the liver shrinks, thus becoming scarred & lumpy; this damage is irreversible and may contribute to liver disease and cancer.

Fibrosis and cirrhosis can take years to grow. To protect the disease from deteriorating, it's important to make behavioral improvements.

Chapter 3. Causes Of Fatty Liver

The liver is the main internal organ in the body, and it is situated on the upper-right of the abdomen. The liver's primary roles are to extract contaminants and process nutrients from food. Before traveling somewhere else in the body, blood from the digestive tract passes into the liver.

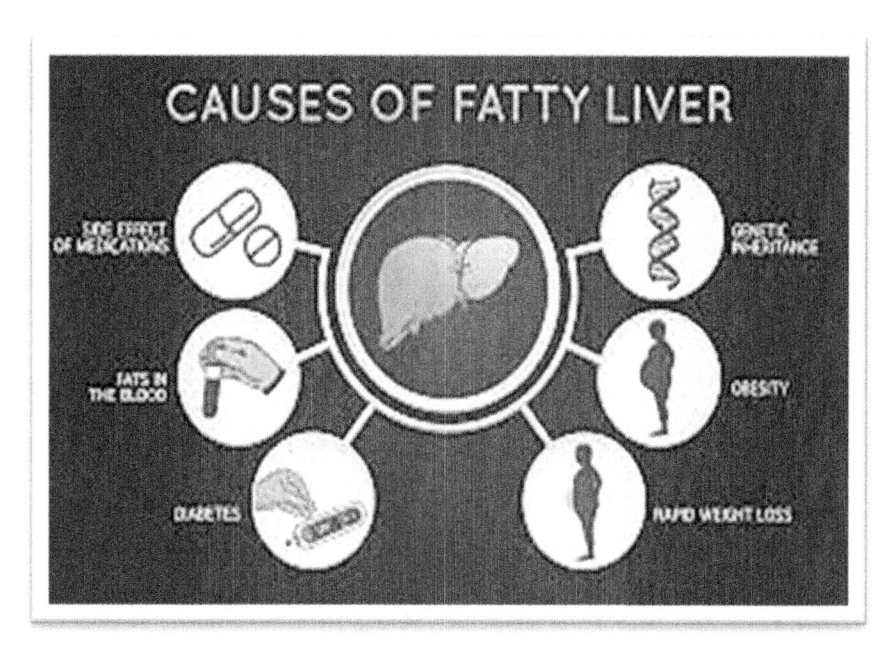

Fatty liver (steatosis) is a popular liver complaint in Western countries, distinguished by excess fat deposition in the liver cells. It affects roughly one out of every ten individuals. While some fat is common in the liver, if fat reaches for more than 10% of the liver's weight, you have fatty liver, which may lead to more severe complications.

While a fatty liver does not cause damage, it may also cause liver inflammation. Steatohepatitis is a disease that causes liver damage. Alcohol addiction is often related to inflammation induced by a fatty liver. Alcoholic steatohepatitis is the medical term for this condition. Non-alcoholic steatohepatitis, or NASH, is the other name for the disease.

Over time, an inflamed liver can become scarred and hardened. Cirrhosis is a dangerous disease that often contributes to liver failure. Cirrhosis is caused by NASH and is one of the main three causes.

3.1 Causes Of Fatty Liver Disease

Excessive calorie intake allows fat to develop in the liver. Too much fat accumulates as the liver does not absorb and break down fats as it should. People with many other diseases, such as obesity, diabetes, or elevated triglycerides, are more likely to develop fatty liver.Fatty liver may also be caused by alcohol consumption, excessive weight loss, and malnutrition. However, even though none of these disorders exist, certain people grow fatty liver.

Fatty Liver Risk Factors:

The majority of fatty liver patients, though not all, are middle-aged & overweight.

The following are the most important risk factors for fatty liver disease:

- overweight
- diabetes
- Elevated triglyceride levels.
- obesity

Metabolic syndrome & fatty liver disease

Many experts now agree that metabolic syndrome, a community of diseases related to an elevated risk of diabetes, cardiac failure, and stroke, plays a central role in fatty liver disease production. The below are signs & symptoms of metabolic syndrome:

- Obesity, particularly around the waistline (abdominal obesity)
- high blood pressure (hypertension)
- Elevated cholesterol levels, such as high triglycerides (a form of blood fat) or low high-density lipoprotein cholesterol (the 'healthy' cholesterol).

- Insulin tolerance, which is a hormone that aids in the regulation of blood sugar levels.

Insulin resistance could be the most significant of these variables in the growth of NASH. Cirrhosis can be caused by a 'second strike' to the liver, including a bacterial infection & hormonal abnormality, and the disease may stay stable for several years with little damage. How does a fatty liver form?

It's unknown how a fatty liver develops. The fat could come from somewhere in the body, or your liver could absorb more fat from your intestine. Another theory is that our liver loses the ability to convert fat into a shape that can be excreted. Fatty foods, on the other hand, do not cause a fatty liver on their own.

3.2 Signs And Symptoms

Who is afflicted by fatty liver disease?

If you do all of the following, you're more likely to have the fatty liver disease:

- Are you Hispanic or Asian in origin?
- Are you a woman who has been through menopause? (A woman whose periods stopped).
- Obesity and a significant volume of excess fat.

- Have high blood pressure, asthma, or cholesterol problem.
- You suffer from obstructive sleep apnea (blocked airway that causes stop and start breathing during sleep).

What are the symptoms of fatty liver disease?

Certain individuals experience fatty liver disorder without experiencing any other health issues. However, the following risk factors raise your odds of catching it:

- Weight or becoming overweight.
- Having diabetes type 2 or insulin resistance.
- Suffering from metabolic syndrome (high cholesterol, insulin resistance, high blood pressure, and high triglyceride levels).
- Take such opioid medicines like amiodarone, diltiazem, tamoxifen, or steroids.

What are the signs and effects of fatty liver?

If the disease progresses towards cirrhosis of the liver, people with fatty liver sometimes experience no signs. If you already have signs, these may involve the following:

Pressure in the right upper side of the abdomen or a sensation of fullness (belly).

- Nausea, a lack of appetite, or a loss of weight.
- Yellowish skin, as well as the whites of the eyes, Called jaundice.
- Abdomen and legs were swollen (edema).
- Excessive exhaustion or mental confusion.
- Deficiency.

3.3 Diagnosis And Tests

How do you know if you have fatty liver disease?

Your doctor could be the first to find fatty liver disorder, and it also has no signs. Increased levels of liver enzymes detected on a blood examination for another disease may be reason for concern. Elevated liver enzymes suggest that the liver has been impaired. Your doctor can order the following tests to make a diagnosis:

- To get an image of the liver, use ultrasound and computed tomography (CT scan).
- A liver biopsy (tissue sample) is conducted to assess the nature of the liver disease.
- FibroScan, a specialized ultrasound that may be used to determine the volume of fat & scar tissue as in the liver instead of a biopsy.

Management And Treatment

What is the cure for fatty liver disease?

There is no clear cure for fatty liver disease. Instead, physicians can consult with you to help you handle the conditions that lead to the illness. They also advise making lifestyle improvements that will help you live a healthier existence. The following is a list of treatments:

- Keeping away from alcoholic drinks.
- Weight loss.
- Taking diabetes, cholesterol, and triglyceride-lowering drugs (fat in the blood).
- In some cases, taking vitamin E and thiazolidinediones (drugs used to cure diabetes such as Actos and Avandia).

Prevention Is Important.

What should be said to stop fatty liver disease?

The easiest way to prevent fatty liver disease is just to keep your general wellbeing in check:

- Achieve a balanced body weight. Lose weight steadily whether you're overweight or obese.
- Exercise daily.

- Limit the alcohol intake to a low.
- Follow the doctor's instructions for taking your drugs.

Prognosis / Outlook

Is it possible to cure fatty liver disease?

The liver has a remarkable capacity to self-repair. It is necessary to reduce liver fat & inflammation and reverse early liver damage, whether you stop drinking or lose weight.

Is fatty liver disorder deadly?

For the most part, the fatty liver disorder does not cause serious complications. However, once it progresses to liver cirrhosis, it may become a much more severe issue. Cirrhosis of the liver, if left unchecked, may lead to liver disease or cancer. Your liver is a vital organ without which you will perish.

Living in Connection

What makes a balanced fatty liver diet?

To lose weight slowly yet gradually, consume a well-balanced diet. The fatty liver disorder may be exacerbated by rapid weight loss. The Mediterranean diet, which is rich in grains, fruits, and healthy fats, is often recommended by doctors. Consult the doctor or a nutritionist with suggestions about how to lose weight safely.

What are some of the questions I can ask my doctor?

- Are there any drugs I'm taking that could induce fatty liver disease?
- What is the magnitude of my liver's damage?
- How long would it take to restore the damage to your liver?
- How can I decide what weight is safe for me?
- Is it possible for me to speak with a nutritionist or attend workshops to hear about healthier eating?

Where do I seek support with an alcohol use disorder?

Consider fatty liver disorder an early warning indicators to help you prevent cirrhosis or liver cancer, which are also lethal liver conditions. And if you don't have any signs of

complications with your liver function right now, it's important to take action to prevent or cure fatty liver disease.

Chapter 4. Problems Due To A Fatty Liver Disease

The fatty liver disease rarely causes serious complications or impairs the liver's ability to act normally. Fatty liver disorder worsens with time for 7% - 30% of those who develop it. It is divided into three stages:

1. Your liver gets inflamed (swollen), causing tissue harm. Steatohepatitis is the name for this point.

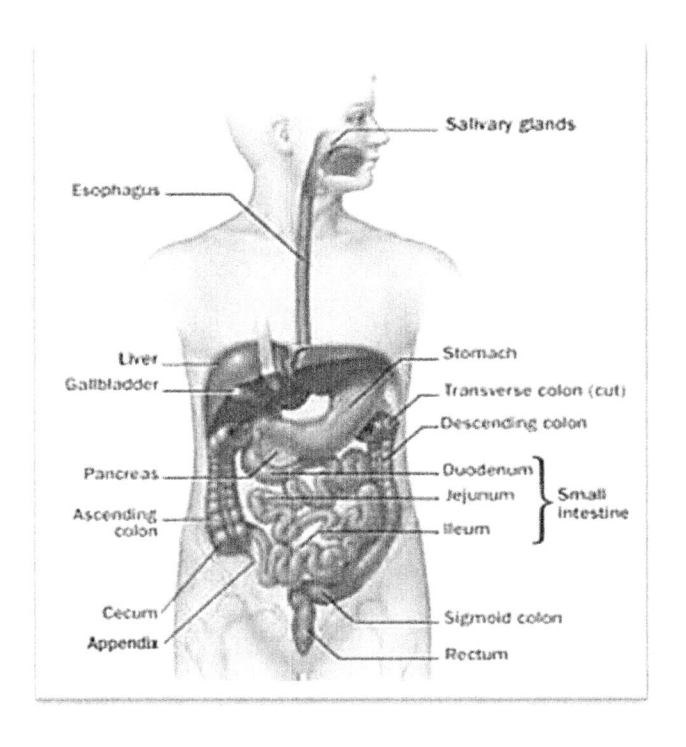

2. When the liver is damaged, scar tissue appears. Fibrosis is the medical name for this disease.

3. Scar tissue eliminates healthy tissue in significant numbers. You have cirrhosis of the liver at this stage.

ARLD-related death rates have increased dramatically in recent decades.

Along with smoking and elevated blood pressure, alcohol consumption is also one of the major causes of mortality in the United Kingdom.

ARLD may trigger life-threatening problems, such as:

4.1 Internal (Variceal) Bleeding

The portal vein usually carries blood from the intestines as well as the spleen to the liver. The regular blood flow through all the liver can become compromised in people with serious liver scarring (cirrhosis). Small arteries in the esophagus and the stomach will then reroute blood from the intestines across the liver.

Varices are enlarged blood vessels that may expand to be very large and swollen. In this case, the spleen can also enlarge. Varices may appear anywhere in the gastrointestinal tract, although the esophagus and stomach are the more frequent locations. Varices will burst due to high pressure and thinning of the walls, causing bleeding in the upper gastrointestinal tract.

Similarly, smaller superficial blood vessels inside the gastrointestinal tract lining may become bloated and ooze blood on occasion. This is known as portal hypertensive gastropathy (until it occurs in the stomach) or colopathy (if it occurs in the colon)

4.2 Toxins Build-Up In The Brain (Encephalopathy)

The word encephalopathy refers to a disorder, damage, or dysfunction of the brain. Encephalopathy may cause a wide variety of effects, from slight memory loss and noticeable personality changes to extreme dementia, epilepsy, paralysis, and death. Encephalopathy is characterized by a change in emotional status that is often followed by physical symptoms (for example, bad coordination of limb movements).

In certain instances, the word encephalopathy is followed by various words that explain the explanation, origin, or specific circumstances that contributed to the patient's brain dysfunction. Anoxic encephalopathy, for example, refers to brain injury caused by a loss of oxygen, whereas hepatic encephalopathy refers to brain malfunction caused by liver failure. Other words either define body disorders or syndromes that result in a complex series of brain dysfunctions. Metabolic encephalopathy &

Wernicke's encephalopathy (Wernicke's syndrome) are two examples. The aim is to introduce the reader to the key types of diseases that come under the general definition of encephalopathy. There are over 150 distinct words that change or initiate "encephalopathy" in the medical literature.

The term "encephalopathy" refers to brain injury or illness. It arises when a shift in the manner your brain operates or a shift in your behavior has an effect on your brain. These shifts result in a shift in your emotional condition, leaving you perplexed and behaving differently than normal.

Encephalopathy is a series of diseases induced for a number of reasons. It's a severe neurological disorder that, if left unchecked, will result in temporary or lasting brain injury.

It's normal to mix up encephalopathy and encephalitis. While the words sound identical, they apply to two separate cases. The brain is bloated or inflamed in encephalitis. On the other hand, encephalopathy is a psychiatric state that may evolve as a consequence of a number of health conditions. Encephalopathy, on the other hand, maybe caused by encephalitis.

Causes and Types

Reversible and permanent encephalopathy are the two primary forms of encephalopathy. The following are examples of reversible causes:

Hepatic encephalopathy. Toxins build up in your bloodstream because your liver becomes unable to extract them from your blood as easily as it can. This makes it impossible for the brain to function properly. It may happen to patients who have cirrhosis or who have taken an excess of acetaminophen or other drugs.

Hashimoto's encephalopathy. This kind is related to Hashimoto's disease, a thyroid disorder. The origin remains unclear, although it's likely that your immune system damages your brain and triggers it to fail.

Metabolic encephalopathy. This occurs while the brain is hampered by some health problems, such as asthma, liver disorder, renal damage, or heart failure. In diabetes, for example, an elevated blood sugar level may cause anxiety and even a coma.

Illnesses of the brain, like encephalitis or meningitis, or infections of the urinary tract. Sepsis, or an overreaction to infection, may result in encephalopathy.

Brain tumors. Toxins such as solvents, medicines, radiation, colors, toxic materials, and other metals may be subjected to over lengthy periods.

Nonconvulsive status epilepticus. This occurs anytime you experience repeated seizures in your head, even though they don't cause any physical effects.

Types of encephalopathy that are irreversible include:

Chronic traumatic encephalopathy. Repeated head injuries affect the brain, resulting in this syndrome. It is also well recognized for its partnerships in high-impact activities such as rugby and boxing.

Hypoxic-ischemic encephalopathy. It occurs anytime the brain does not get enough oxygen, resulting in brain damage. After cardiac arrest, drug overdose, carbon monoxide poisoning, or near-drowning, it will happen.

4.3 Abdomen Fluid Accumulation (Ascites) Associated Kidney Failure

The term ascites comes from the Greek word askos, which means bag or sac. The state of pathologic fluid accumulation inside the abdominal cavity is referred to as ascites. Depending on their menstrual cycle level, stable males have little to no intraperitoneal fluid, whereas women may have as many as 20 ml.

ASCITES
LAPAROCENTESIS

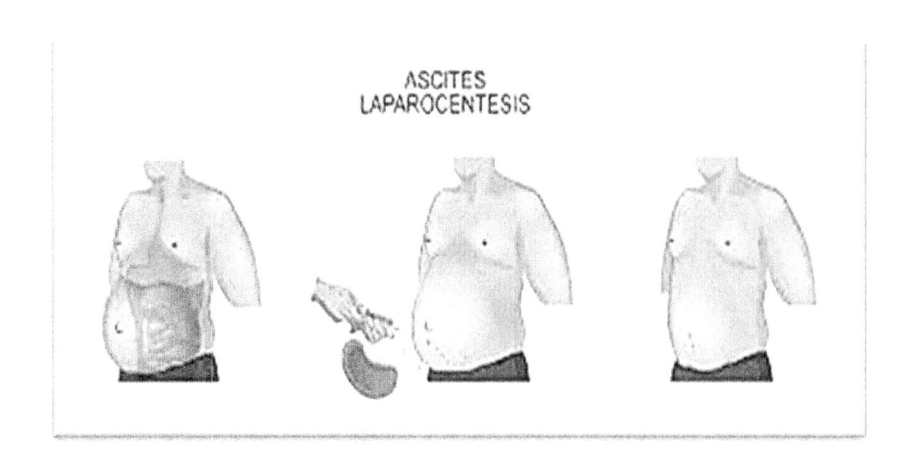

Ascites are a syndrome in which blood accumulates in the abdominal cavity. Ascites may be uncomfortable if it is serious. You could be unable to move about freely as a result of the issue. Ascites may lead to an infection in the abdominal cavity. Fluid may even penetrate the chest and encircle your lungs. It's tough to breathe because of this.

Ascites are a disease in which more than 25 milliliters (mL) of fluid builds up within the abdomen. When the liver ceases functioning correctly, ascites develop. Fluid occupies the gap between the stomach lining and the organs as the liver malfunctions.

The three-year survival rate is 50%, according to clinical recommendations released in the Journal of Hepatology in 2010. Consult the doctor right away whether you are having ascites symptoms.

What causes ascites?

Ascites are the result of a sequence of incidents. The most frequent source of ascites is liver cirrhosis. Cirrhosis induces a blockage of the movement of blood into the liver. The strain in the key vein (the portal vein), which carries blood from the digestive organs to the liver, increases due to the blockage. Portal hypertension is the medical term for this disorder. As portal hypertension progresses, ascites develop. The kidneys are unable to remove sufficiently sodium (salt) from the body by urine. When the body cannot rid itself of salt, fluids build up in the liver, resulting in ascites.

What are the complications of the ascites stage?

Abdominal pain, discomfort & difficulty breathing: If there is so much blood in the stomach cavity, this may cause complications. This will make it difficult for a patient to chew, walk, or do any everyday tasks.

Infection: Bacteria could infect the fluids that accumulate in the stomach as a consequence of ascites. Spontaneous bacterial peritonitis is the term for what occurs as this happens. Fever and stomach pain are the two prominent signs. Taking samples from the abdominal cavity, as mentioned above, is normally used to render the diagnosis. Spontaneous bacterial peritonitis is a critical disease that necessitates IV antibiotic therapy. Once you've recovered from this infection, you'll continue to take oral antibiotics for the rest of your life to prevent the infection from coming again.

Fluid in the lungs: Hepatic hydrothorax is the medical term for this disease. The lungs are packed with stomach fat (normally on the right side). Cough, shortness of breath, hypoxemia (lack of oxygen in the blood), and chest pain are all symptoms of this condition. The easiest way to manage hepatic hydrothorax is to remove the abdominal ascites through the paracentesis.

Kidney failure: Cirrhosis of the liver that worsens may contribute to kidney failure. Hepatorenal syndrome is the psychiatric name for this disease. While it is uncommon, it is a dangerous illness that may lead to kidney failure.

Symptoms of ascites

- Weight gain
- Swelling in the abdomen
- Sense of heaviness
- Sense of fullness
- Bloating

- Nausea or indigestion
- Hemorrhoids
- Swelling in lower legs
- Vomiting
- Shortness of breath

4.4 Liver Cancer

Liver cancer develops as the DNA of liver cells improves (mutates). The DNA of a cell is the substance that contains the guidance for all of your body's chemical processes. DNA mutations cause changes in these instructions. Consequently, cells can develop out of control which eventually forms a tumor, which is a group of cancerous cells.

In certain cases, such as with untreated hepatitis diseases, the origin of liver cancer is recognized. However, liver cancer may occur in individuals with no underlying illnesses, and the cause is unknown.

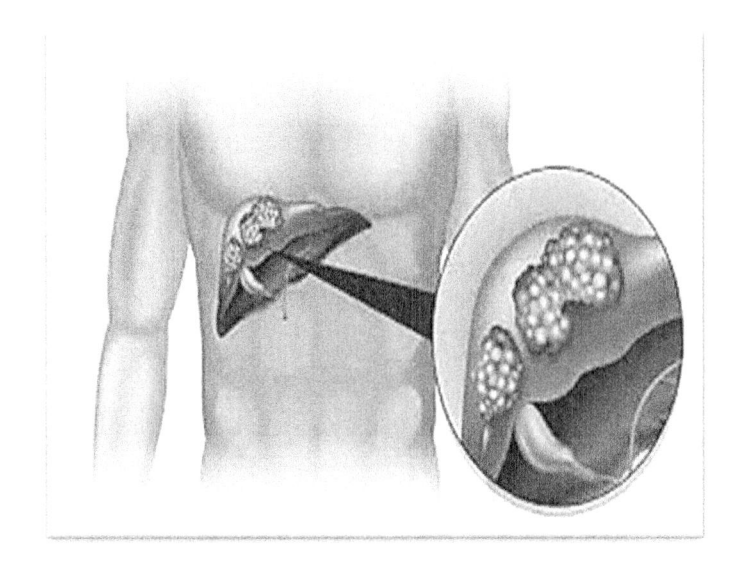

Cancer that starts in the cells of the liver is known as liver cancer. The liver is a broad organ that lies in your body's upper right section, under your diaphragm, just above your stomach.

The liver will develop a variety of cancers. Hepatocellular carcinoma is the most prevalent type of liver cancer, and it starts with the primary group of liver cells (hepatocyte). Other forms of liver cancer are much less common, like intrahepatic cholangiocarcinoma and hepatoblastoma.

The spread of cancer to the liver is more likely than cancer that starts with the liver cells. Metastatic cancer, rather than liver cancer, starts in some part of the body, such as the colon, lung, or breast, and eventually progresses to the liver. Metastatic colon cancer, for example, is a form of cancer that starts in the colon and extends to the liver.

Main symptoms of liver cancer

There may be no signs, or they may be impossible to identify in people with liver cancer.

If liver cancer begins there in the liver (primary liver cancer) or travels from another section of the body, the signs are the same (secondary liver cancer).

The below are some of the signs and symptoms of liver cancer:

- You might have itchy ears, darker pee, and paler poo than normal if your skin or whites' eyes turn yellow (jaundice).
- Loss in appetite or weight loss without attempting to do so
- A sense of exhaustion or a lack of resources
- Feeling unwell in general or developing flu-like symptoms
- A lump in the stomach on the right side
- Some signs and symptoms that may impact the digestion include:
- Being sick or feeling bad

- Pain on your right shoulder or the right side of your tummy

- Indigestion signs include getting satisfied quite soon after eating.

- A swollen stomach that is unrelated to when you eat

4.5 Increased Vulnerability To Infection

Immuno-compromised cancer patients are more susceptible to contamination for a variety of reasons. While there is some correlation between predisposing factors and some infections, they are linked to a distinct group of infections. Predisposing conditions may arise in the same patient, broadening the number of diseases that could develop. Recognizing these aspects allows the intelligent clinician to make a reliable diagnosis of the future pathogen(s) in a given patient or environment and to begin empiric therapy as soon as possible. The most

prominent defects in host protection systems are related to multiple cancers and the infections linked to such defects.

Chapter 5. Fatty Liver Disease Diet

That is correct. If your liver could talk to you, it will say: "I'm working hard, trying my utmost to turn what you eat & drink into energy and nutrients, even though you can't see it tucked under your rib cage." Hey, I'm your filter, too! I'm attempting to extract possibly dangerous chemicals from the body. So, won't you at the very least help me?"

Isn't it strange that a communicating liver exists? Your liver, on the other side, does interact with you.

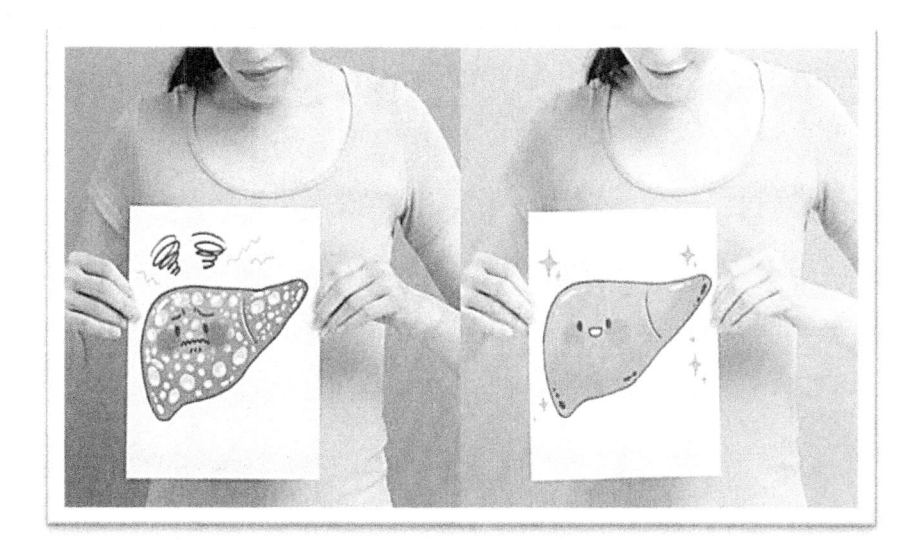

Your liver "tells" you that you're doing a decent job if you follow a balanced diet. You get the warning that the liver is sufficiently effective, and you are in outstanding physical condition if your overall health is perfect.

Your stomach, on the other side, is helpless if you don't watch what you eat. Your liver is actually under threat when you eat unhealthy or fried foods and a lot of salt.

Your liver cannot assist you until you assist it. As a consequence, the liver struggles from cancer, as well as other organ-related problems. Maintaining a healthy weight is, of course, important. Exercise daily, in addition to maintaining a balanced lifestyle.

For nutrition and insulation, the liver stores fat in several places. Fat is found as part of the liver. High-fat content in the liver, on the other side, may suggest fatty liver disease. For this liver disease, lifestyle modifications are the first line of protection.

The fatty liver disorder can be classified into two categories: alcoholic and nonalcoholic. The fatty liver disorder is often a risk in pregnancy.

The liver is damaged by fatty liver disease, which prevents it from absorbing contaminants and processing bile for digestion. When the liver cannot conduct these functions properly, an individual is at risk of having other health issues in their body.

The fatty liver disorder may be managed with dietary modifications and daily exercise. Any patients, though, will continue to see a specialist for further care.

We recommend some items to use in a fatty liver disease diet and foods to avoid in this report.

5.1 Foods For A Fatty Liver

Garlic can help people with the fatty liver disease lose weight.

A fatty liver disease diet can consist of a large range of foods.

A healthy way to start is by lowering calorie consumption and consuming high fiber, fresh foods. Complex carbohydrates, fiber, and protein-rich foods may provide long-lasting nutrition and encourage satiety.

Foods that help the body regenerate its cells or reduce inflammation are equally essential.

Some people adopt particular eating plans, such as the Mediterranean diet or a plant-based diet. A dietitian will also help a person create a tailored diet plan that is suitable for their needs, symptoms, and current health status.

In addition to these general recommendations, certain diets can be more useful to fatty liver disease people. Among these foods are:

Garlic

Garlic is a popular ingredient in many diets, and it can help individuals with fatty liver disease. According to a 2016 report published in Advanced Biomedical Research, garlic powder supplements tend to help people with fatty liver disease lose weight and overweight.

Garlic powdered supplements Trusted Source not only bring spice to cooking, but they've also been shown in tests to support people for fatty liver disease lose weight and overweight.

Omega-3 fatty acids

In individuals with nonalcoholic fatty liver disease, eating omega-3 fatty acids increases liver fat and lipoprotein (HDL) cholesterol levels, according to a 2016 study of existing studies.

While further study is needed to validate this result, foods rich in omega-3 fatty acids can reduce liver fat. Among these foods are:

- Salmon
- flaxseed
- sardines
- walnuts

Coffee

According to studies, coffee consumers with fatty liver disorder have fewer liver damage than people who do not consume this caffeinated product. Caffeine reduces the level of excess liver enzymes in individuals at risk of developing liver failure.

For certain individuals, consuming coffee is a morning routine. People with fatty liver disease, on the other hand, can recover from it beyond a release of energy.

Decaffeinated coffee minimized liver damage & inflammation in mice fed a high-fat, fructose, and cholesterol diet, according to a 2019 animal report.

Mouse research published the same year yielded identical findings. According to the researchers, coffee lowered the amount of fat that developed in the mice's livers and changed how their bodies metabolized energy.

Broccoli Greens

People with fatty liver disorder benefit from consuming many whole vegetables. On the other hand, broccoli is a vegetable that people with the fatty liver disorder can have in their diet.

Broccoli has been shown in mouse to help prevent fat

accumulation in the liver. Adding more vegetables to the diet, such as lettuce, Brussels sprouts, and kale, will also assist in weight reduction. Try the vegetarian chili recipe from the Canadian Liver Foundation, which allows you to slash calories without losing taste.

According to a 2016 animal report released in The Journal of Diet, long-term intake of broccoli helped avoid fat accumulation in murine livers.

Human studies are also required, according to the researchers. Early studies into the impact of broccoli intake upon this development of fatty liver disease, on the other hand, seem to be encouraging.

Tofu

Soy protein, which is present in foods like tofu, decreased fat production in the liver in a rat study at the University of Illinois. Tofu is also high in protein and low in fat.

Fish for inflammation

Omega-3 fatty acids are abundant in fatty fish like salmon, sardines, tuna & trout. Omega-3 fatty acids may help remove liver fat. A Trustworthy Source for Minimizing Inflammation Source you can trust. Try this low-fat teriyaki halibut recipe, which comes highly recommended by the Canadian Liver Foundation.

Oatmeal for energy

Carbohydrates from whole grains, such as oatmeal, provide nutrients to the body. Their fiber quality keeps you fuller for longer, which will help you stay on track with your weight.

Avocado to protect the liver

According to studies, avocados are rich in good fats and contain chemicals that can help prevent liver harm. They're also abundant in fiber, which will help you drop weight. Fatty Liver Diet Review recommends this refreshing avocado & mushroom salad.

Milk & other low-fat dairies

According to a 2011 study in rats, dairy is rich in whey protein, which can shield the liver from more damage.

Sunflower seeds for antioxidants

Vitamin E, an antioxidant that can shield the liver from more damage, is plentiful in these nutty-tasting seeds.

Olive oil usage for weight control

Omega-3 fatty acids are abundant in this helpful oil. It's a better alternative to butter, margarine, or shortening for food. Olive oil is found to help regulate weight and lower liver enzyme levels, according to Research.

Grapefruit

Grapefruit is rich in antioxidants, which tend to defend the liver naturally. Naringenin and naringin are the two primary antioxidants present in Grapefruit.

Both have been shown in animal research to better shield the liver from damage.

Grapefruit's antioxidant properties are believed to arise in two ways: by reducing inflammation and protecting cells.

These antioxidants have also been shown in studies to aid in the prevention of hepatic fibrosis, a dangerous disease in which unnecessary connective tissue develops in the liver. Chronic inflammation is usually the cause of this.

Furthermore, naringenin reduced the volume of fat in the liver also raised the number of fat-burning enzymes in mice fed a high-fat diet, which may help deter extra fat from gathering.

Finally, naringin has been shown to enhance the capacity to metabolize alcohol & counteract some of the toxic effects of alcohol in rats.

Grapefruit or grapefruit juice, rather than its constituents, has not yet been tested for its influence. Furthermore, nearly all experiments on grapefruit antioxidants have been carried out on livestock.

On the other side, Grapefruit tends to be a safe way to maintain the liver balanced by avoiding degradation and inflammation.

Blueberries and cranberries

Anthocyanin, the antioxidants that lend berries their distinctive colors, are present in both blueberries and cranberries. They've even been attributed to a variety of health benefits.

Whole cranberries & blueberries and their extracts or juices have been shown in many animal trials to help maintain liver health.

The liver was protected from damage after 21 days of eating these fruits. Blueberries have tended to improve immune cell activity and antioxidant enzymes.

Another research discovered that antioxidants present in blueberries delayed the growth of lesions and fibrosis, or scar tissue forming, in livers of the rats.

Furthermore, in test-tube tests, the blueberry extract has been shown to prevent human liver cancer cells' development. More study is required to see whether this impact can be repeated in the human body.

Making these berries a daily part of your diet will ensure that your liver gets the antioxidants it requires to stay safe.

Grapes

Grapes, especially red or purple grapes, contain several plant compounds that are beneficial to health. Resveratrol is the most well-known, and it has a host of health benefits.

Grapes and grape juice are beneficial to the liver in several animal trials.

According to studies, they have been shown to have a variety of benefits, including reducing inflammation, preventing injury, and can antioxidant levels.

According to a limited report, supplementing with grape seed extract about three months helped increase liver function in humans with NAFLD.

However, since grape seed extract would be a distilled form, you can not experience the same outcomes as if you consumed entire grapes. Before grape seed extracts for the liver could be prescribed, further research is required.

Despite this, a broad body of research from animal and human research shows that grapes are a liver-friendly product.

Prickly pear

Opuntia ficus-indica, or prickly pear in scientific terms, is a common edible cactus. Its fruit & juice are the most common.

It's been used in western medicine for a long time as a remedy for:

- Ulcers
- Fatigue
- Liver Disease
- Wounds

This plant's extract was shown to help alleviate hangover effects in 55 people in a 2004 trial.

There was less fatigue, dry throat, and a loss of appetite among the participants. Therefore, they were half as likely to get a bad hangover if they took the extract before consuming alcohol, which the liver detoxifies.

The researchers concluded that these results were attributed to a decline in inflammation, which is normal after consuming alcohol.

Another research in mice showed that while prickly pear

extract was eaten with a pesticide considered to be toxic to the liver, it tended to normalize enzyme and cholesterol levels. Subsequent experiments produced identical findings.

More recently, a rat analysis was conducted to see whether prickly pear juice, instead of the extract, successfully mitigated the harmful effects of alcohol.

The juice was shown to help minimize the level of oxidative damage and harm to the liver after alcohol intake and maintain antioxidant and inflammation levels constant.

More human trials are required, with prickly pear fruit & juice rather than extract being used. Nonetheless, tests to date have shown that prickly pear has favorable effects on the liver.

Beetroot juice

Beetroot juice includes nitrates and betalains, which can protect the heart and reduce oxidative damage & inflammation.

It's fair to conclude that consuming beets has similar health consequences. The bulk of reports, however, use beet juice. Beet juice may be made at home or purchased at a supermarket or online.

Beetroot juice has been shown to help minimize oxidative damage & inflammation in the liver and improve natural detoxification enzymes in many rat studies.

Although animal tests seem positive, no human studies have been undertaken.

Beetroot juice has also been seen to provide other health benefits in animal tests, confirmed in human studies. More research is required, however, to validate the effects of beetroot juice on human liver health.

Cruciferous vegetables

Cruciferous foods, such as Brussels sprouts, broccoli, and mustard greens, are rich in fiber and have a distinct flavor. They're even rich in plant compounds that are safe for you.

Brussels sprouts & broccoli sprout extract have been shown in animal tests to increase detoxification enzyme levels and shield the liver from damage.

According to a report, this influence was observed in human liver cells even after Brussels sprouts were fried.

Mice feeding broccoli produced less tumors, and fatty liver disease than mice fed a control diet, according to a 2016 report.

The number of human studies is limited. However, cruciferous vegetables seem to be a promising food for liver health so far.

To make a delicious and nutritious dish, gently roast them with garlic & lemon juice or balsamic vinegar.

Green tea

Tea has been used to treat a variety of ailments for thousands of years.

Green tea can help lower fat levels in the blood and throughout the body, according to a study published in World Journal of Gastroenterology in 2015. One experiment found that people who consume 5–9 cups of green tea a day had lower amounts of fat in their liver.

Green tea has been seen to help prevent fat absorption, although the evidence isn't yet definitive. Green tea is being studied to see how it will help decrease fat storage in the liver, increasing liver function. Green tea, on the other side, has various advantages, varying from cholesterol suppression to sleep help.

Green tea contains antioxidants, including catechin, which can aid in the treatment of fatty liver disease.

Walnuts

Although all tree nuts are beneficial to a healthy diet, walnuts are particularly rich in omega-3 fatty acids and can help people from fatty liver disease.

Omega-3 fatty acids are found in these nuts. According to research, eating walnuts improves liver function measures in people with fatty liver disorder.

Walnut consumption increased liver function test outcomes in individuals with nonalcoholic fatty liver disorder, according to a 2015 study.

Soy or whey protein

Both soy and whey protein were found to decrease fat production in the liver in a study published in the journal Nutrients in 2019. One research in the analysis found that eating 55 grams of whey protein a day for four weeks reduced liver fat by 20% in obese women. Soy protein includes isoflavones, which are antioxidants that can increase insulin response and lower fat levels in the body.

Fatty fish

Omega-3 fatty acids, found in fatty fish, are beneficial fats that help suppress inflammation and have been linked to a reduced risk of heart disease.

Omega 3 fatty acids were shown to help individuals with nonalcoholic fatty liver disorder or nonalcoholic steatohepatitis reduces their liver fat and triglycerides in a 2016 study.

Although eating omega-3-rich fatty fish seems to be good for your liver, it's not the only thing to think about.

The ratio of omega-3 to omega-6 fatty acids is also essential.

Most Americans consume more omega-6 fats, which are present in many plant oils than is recommended. A high omega-6 to omega-3 ratio may contribute to the production of liver disease.

As a consequence, it's a smart idea to cut down on omega-6 fats as well.

5.2 Foods To Avoid

One approach to treat the fatty liver disorder is to eat more healthy foods. Therefore, individuals with this disorder need to prevent or restrict their use of many other foods.

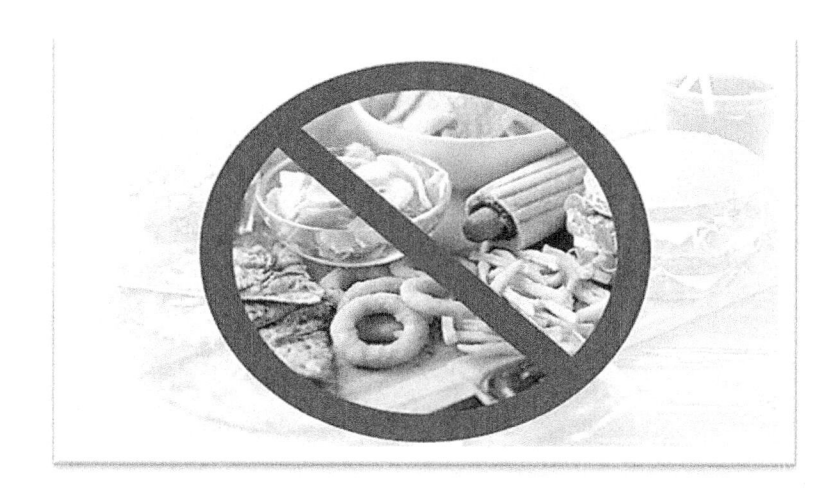

It's easy to believe that "fat" is the main cause of NAFLD, but it's really sugar and carbs. While avoiding saturated fat is critical for optimal health and weight loss, lowering carb consumption would result in the most significant change in your condition.

Alcohol

The most frequent source of fatty liver disease is alcohol. Alcohol has an effect on the liver, causing fatty liver disease or other liver disorders, including cirrhosis.

When you have NAFLD, one of the most critical items to stop is alcohol. Alcohol may not only worsen fatty liver disorder; however, it may often exacerbate an established illness.

If you have fatty liver syndrome due to excessive drinking, you can not drink at all. It has the potential to cause more severe liver injury. If you have NAFLD, you can be able to have a drink every other month, just not more than that. Consult the physician first.

If you have fatty liver disorder, you can cut down on alcohol or exclude it entirely from your diet.

Sugar and added sugars

Sugar, including naturally occurring sugars like fruit juice & honey, should be minimized in some form.

Added sugars raise blood sugar levels which may lead to a rise in liver fat.

Sugar is typically applied to sweets, ice cream, as well as sweetened beverages like soda and fruit drinks by producers.

Packaged snacks, baked products, and store-bought tea and coffee have added sugars. Some carbohydrates, like fructose & corn syrup, can be avoided to reduce liver fat.

Refined grains

White bread, white pasta, or white rice both contain processed and refined grains. The fiber in these heavily refined grains has been lost, which may cause blood sugar to rise when the body turns them down.

In a 2015 survey of 73 people with nonalcoholic fatty liver

disease, it was discovered that those who ate less processed carbohydrates have a lower incidence of metabolic syndrome, which is a set of risk factors that raises the risk of cardiac disease and stroke.

People may conveniently substitute legumes, or whole-wheat, potatoes, and whole-grain substitutes for processed grains.

Salt

Maintain a sodium consumption of less than 1500 milligrams per day. You will retain water weight if you consume so much salt.

Fried or salty foods

Excessive consumption of fried or salty foods would raise calorie intake and increase the likelihood of weight gain. The fatty liver disorder is often triggered by obesity.

Using additional herbs and spices to a meal to flavor it without adding salt is a perfect way to do so. Instead of frying, people will normally bake or steam their rice.

Fries, candy, chicken wings, and donuts are rich in fat and sugar. Blood sugar levels can increase as a result of these diets, which is a leading factor to NAFLD.

Saturated fat

Saturated fats, such as those used in red meat and butter, can be avoided in favor of healthier fats such as olive, avocado, or cold-pressed nut oils.

Poultry

Owing to its high-fat content of chicken wings and thighs, poultry is only recommended if it is a slice of white meat. If you want to consume white chicken meat, be sure to remove the skin and fat.

Refined carbs

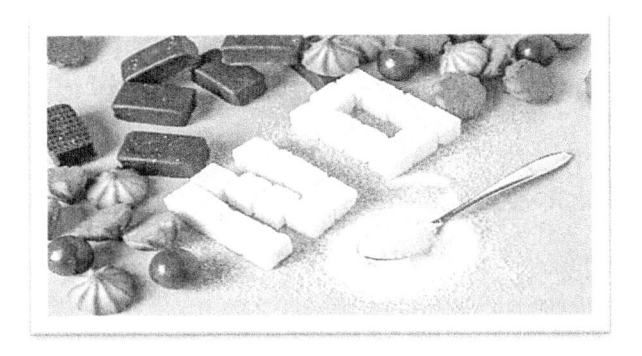

Whole grain substitutes such as quinoa, whole wheat flour, and black bean pasta can be substituted for white carbohydrates such as white bread and pasta.

Meat

Saturated fat consumption raises the volume of fat which builds up across organs, including the liver, according to a research published in 2019. Saturated fats are high in pork, beef, and deli meats, which a person having fatty liver disease should avoid.

Substitutes include lean meats, pork, tofu, and tempeh. On the other hand, wild, oily fish could be the better option since they often have omega-3 fatty acids.

Chapter 6. Recipes for Nourishing the Fatty Liver

The liver is an amazing organ with incredible regenerative abilities. Along with the intestines, pancreas, and gallbladder, it aids absorption, clears our organs, and aids in metabolizing drugs and detoxifying chemicals. According to conventional Chinese medicine, the liver carries qi, or essential energy, through our muscles and joints.

Our liver, together with the kidneys, is a big toxin filtering mechanism. Our hormones, vision, hair, and skin are all affected by the liver. The liver is considered by the Chinese to be the body's "General," a commanding officer from whom all of our wellbeing or illness stems.

Because of unhealthy foods, medications of all types, smoking, and diets high in animal products, modern habits put a significant strain on the liver. According to five-element food, the wood element, liver, is nurturing to the wood element, liver, which is a great choice for planning a meal to preserve and help the liver function.

6.1 Breakfast Recipes For Fatty Liver

1. Tomato & Watermelon Salad

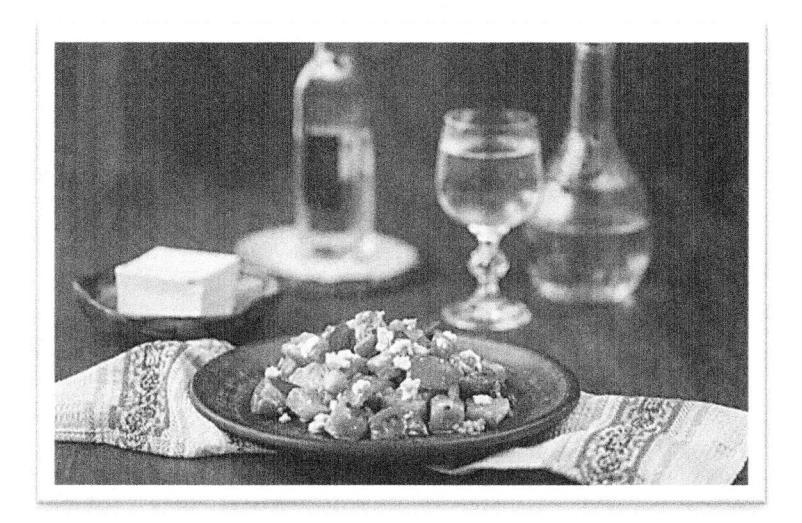

Prep Time + Cook Time: 5 Minutes

Servings: 2

Ingredients

- 1 tbsp of olive oil
- 1 tbsp of red wine vinegar
- ¼ tsp of chili flakes
- 1 tbsp of chopped mint
- 120g / ⅝ of cup chopped tomatoes
- ½ watermelon, chunks
- 50g / ⅔ cup of feta cheese, crumbled

Instructions

To create the dressing, whisk together the oil, vinegar, chili flakes, mint, and season to taste.

In a mixing bowl, combine the tomatoes and watermelon. Pour the dressing over the salad, top with the feta, and serve.

2. Banana Yogurt Pots

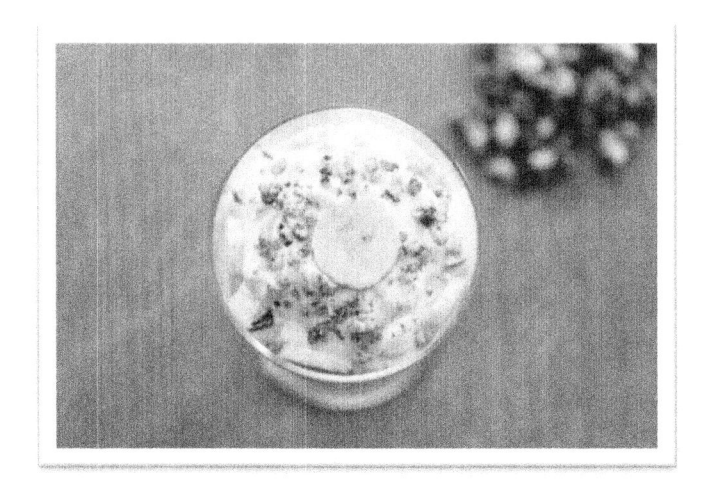

Prep time + Cook Time: 5 minutes

Serving: 2

Ingredients

- ⅞ cup of Greek yogurt
- 2 tbsp of walnuts, toasted & chopped
- Two bananas, sliced and chunks

Instructions

In the bottom of a bottle, pour some of the yogurts. Repeat with a layer of banana and yogurt till the glass is full.

3. Healthy Oatmeal Breakfast

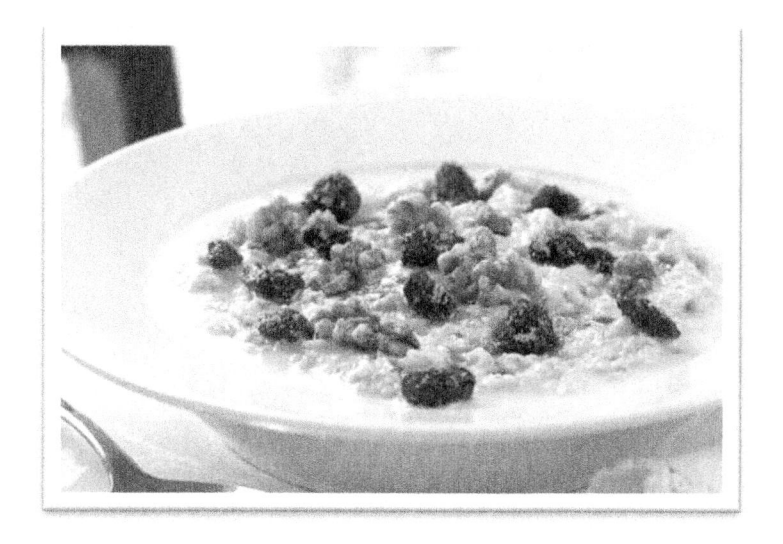

Prep time + Cook Time: 5 minutes

Serving: 2

Ingredients

- ½ cup of quick oats or steel rolled oats
- Fist-full of raisins (if possible, organic) – approx. ½ cup
- 1 tsp. clover honey
- 1 tsp. ground cinnamon.

- 1 tsp. pure maple syrup
- 1 cup of water (steel rolled oats) or 1 cup of boiling water (quick oats)

Instructions

Steel rolled oats – prepare per label directions.

When steel-rolled oats are finished cooking, add the remaining ingredients.

Mix thoroughly and enjoy.

4. Non-Dairy Cornmeal Breakfast

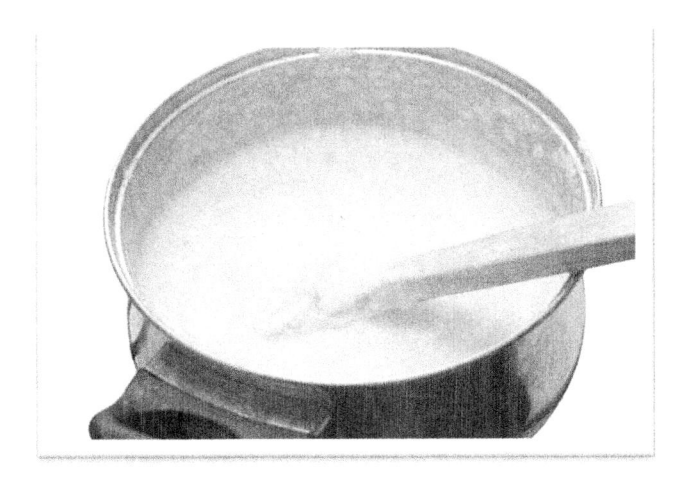

Prep time + Cook Time: 5 minutes

Servings: 2

Ingredients

- 1-1/2 cups of unsweetened almond milk

- 1 cup of corn meal (prefer corn grits)
- 2 cups of cold water
- Salt, grape seed oil & pure maple syrup (very little amounts of each – just to taste)

Instructions

In a medium saucepan, pour the almond milk. Switch the heat on.

Combine corn meal and cool water in a mixing bowl. Stir this paste into the saucepan thoroughly.

Bring to a simmer over high flame, stirring regularly. Reduce the heat and stir often to avoid sticking.

Remove from heat as thickened and season with salt, grape-seed oil, and pure maple syrup for a taste.

5. **Blueberry Oats Bowl**

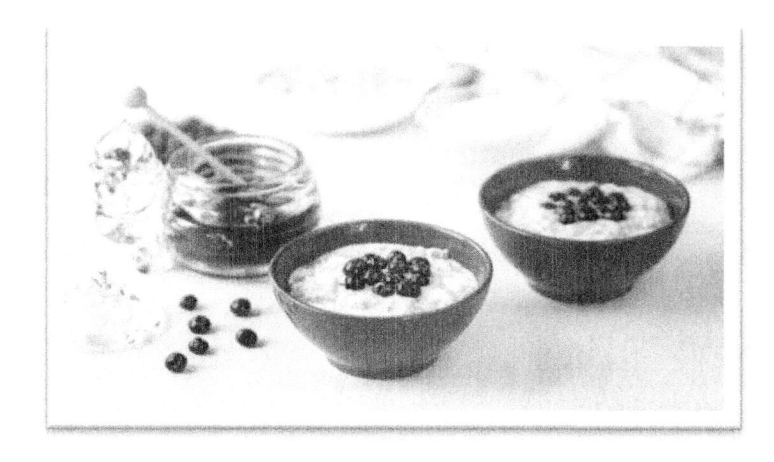

Prep time + Cook time: 10 minutes

Servings: 2

Ingredients

- ⅔ cup of porridge oats
- 175g blueberries
- ⅗ cup of Greek yogurt
- 1 tsp of honey

Instructions

In a pan, combine the oats and 400ml of water. For around 2 minutes, heat and swirl. Take the pan off the heat and stir about a third of the yogurt.

Combine the blueberries, sugar, and 1 tbsp of water in a tub. Gently poach the blueberries until they are soft.

Place the leftover yogurt and blueberries on top of the porridge in cups.

6. Spinach Feta Breakfast Wraps

Prep time + Cook time: 50 minutes

Servings: 4

Ingredients

- Ten large eggs

- 1/2 pound baby spinach (about 5 cups)
- Four whole-wheat tortillas (burrito-sized, about 9 inches)
- 1/2 pint of cherry or grape tomatoes, cut halved
- 4 ounces of feta cheese, crumbled
- Olive oil or butter
- Pepper
- Salt

Instructions

Whisk the eggs in a large mixing bowl before the whites & yolks are fully mixed. Over medium flame, melt sufficiently butter or olive oil so cover the bottom of a large skillet. Pour in the eggs until the butter has melted or the oil has heated up, and regularly mix before the eggs are fried. Shift to a large plate for cool at room temperature after adding a pinch of salt & a generous quantity of black pepper.

Replace the skillet over medium heat after rinsing or wiping it clean, then apply another pat of oil or butter. Cook, often stirring, till the spinach has wilted slightly. Cooked spinach can be laid out on a large plate for cool at room temperature.

On a work surface, place a tortilla. Place a quarter of the tomatoes, spinach, eggs, and feta cheese down the tortilla center and tie tightly. Go on for the three remaining tortillas in the same manner. Freeze the wraps in such a gallon zip-top container before you're able to consume them. Cover the burritos in aluminum foil if freezing for longer than a week to avoid freezer burn. Microwave on full for 2 minutes to reheat.

7. Fluffy Vegan Waffles

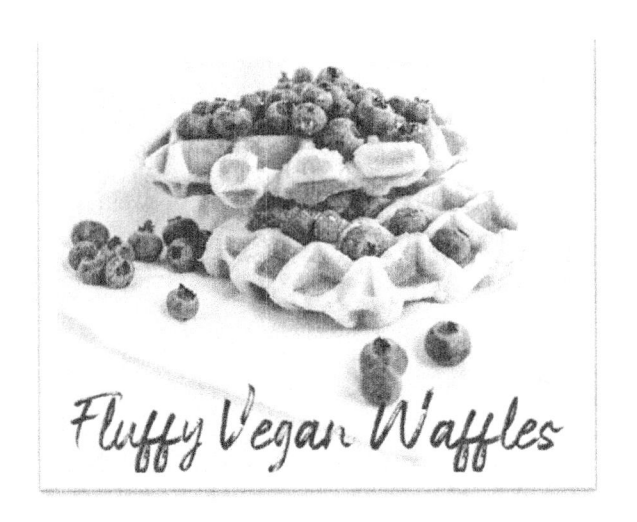

Prep time + Cook time: 25 minutes

Servings: 6

Ingredients

- 1 1/2 cups of coconut milk or unsweetened almond (room temperature)

- 1 Tbsp of baking powder
- 2 cups of all-purpose flour
- 1/2 tsp of baking soda
- 1/2 tsp of salt
- 2 Tbsp of brown sugar maple syrup
- 1/2 tsp of alcohol-free vanilla extract
- 1/4 cup of melted coconut oil

Five add-ins to try optional (not though at the same time):

- 1 tsp of pumpkin pie spice
- 1 tsp of cinnamon
- 1/4 cup of cocoa powder
- 1/4 cup of dairy-free chocolate chips
- 1 tsp of lemon zest – topped with blueberries is delicious!

Directions

Combine the milk and vinegar in a medium bowl and set aside for 5 minutes. Buttermilk would be generated as a result of this.

In a separate, big mixing cup, stir together the dry ingredients: flour, baking powder, salt, and baking soda.

Add the sugar or syrup, coconut oil, and vanilla to the buttermilk. To mix, stir all together.

Pour the wet ingredients into the dry ingredients and stir just enough to blend them. Over mixing can result in lumps in the batter.

Allow 10 minutes for the batter to rest.

Preheat your waffle iron to moderate flame and your oven to 200 ° Fahrenheit.

Using a nonstick spray, lightly coat the bottom and sides of the waffle iron.

Fill the waffle iron halfway with batter. Close the waffle iron softly and cook until no steam escapes and the waffle is lightly browned and fresh, around 4-5 minutes.

Remove the waffles from the pan and hold them warm on a baking sheet within your preheated oven before all of the waffles are done.

Serve with your preferred syrup, spread, or fruit right away!

8. Best Homemade Granola

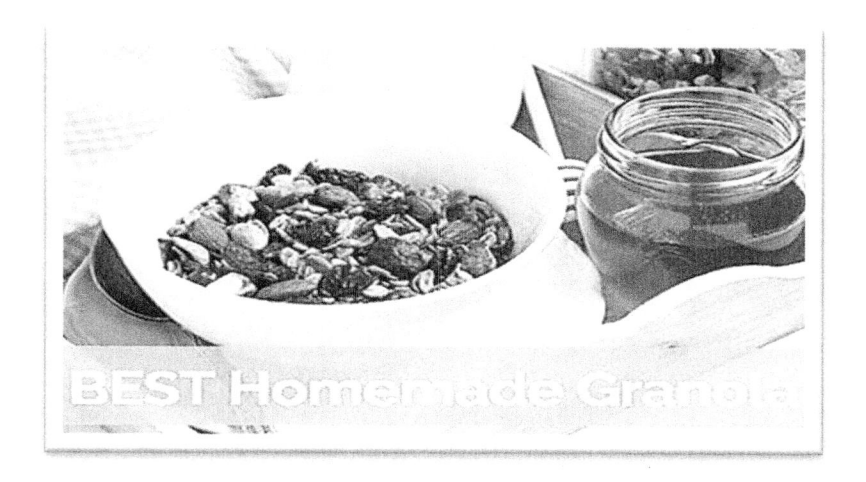

Prep time + Cook time: 25 minutes

Servings: 6

Ingredients

- 4 cups of organic rolled oats
- 1/2 cup of hazelnuts chopped
- 1/2 cup of slivered chopped almonds
- 2 tbsp of seeds (flax)
- 3 tbsp of sugar brown
- 1 cup of coconut shredded
- 1/2 tsp of cinnamon
- 1/2 tsp of salt
- 1/4 tsp of nutmeg

- 1/3 cup of applesauce
- 1/3 cup of apple cider or apple juice or
- 1 cup of cranberries dried or dried chopped fruit
- 1/3 cup of honey

Instructions

Preheat the oven to 300 degrees Fahrenheit. Combine the oats, nuts, coconut, brown sugar, cinnamon, flax seeds, nutmeg, and salt in a large mixing bowl.

In a mixing cup, combine the applesauce, honey with apple juice.

Pour the pure liquid over the oat mixture, then stir through a wooden spoon to cover all of the oats and nuts.

Spread the granola on a wide sheet pan lined by the parchment paper and bake for 30-40 minutes, stirring with a spatula every 10 minutes until the combination turns a nice, light golden brown.

Remove the granola from the oven, then let it cool entirely before stirring it. Stir in the cranberries.

Granola may be kept in the refrigerator for many weeks in an airtight jar or plastic bag. It can be eaten plain, with cheese, or with almond milk.

9. Easter Brunch Egg Baskets

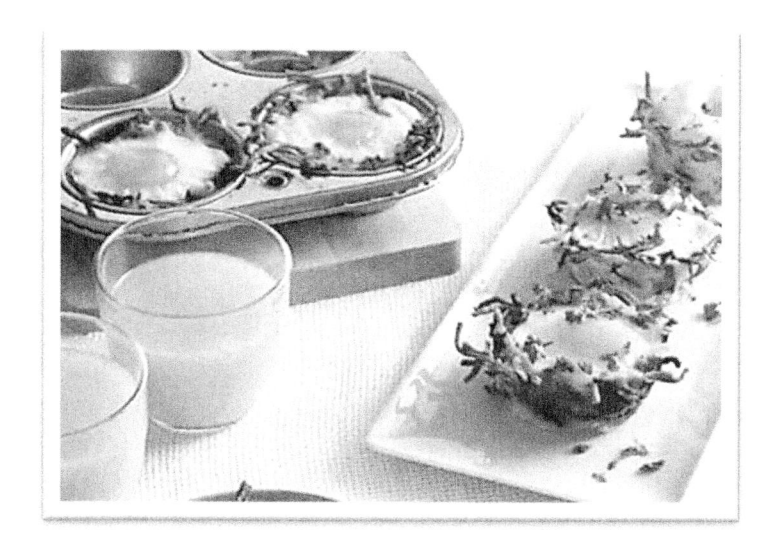

Prep time + Cook time: 25 minutes

Servings: 6

Ingredients

Egg Potato Basket

- 1/4 cup of refrigerated hash brown shredded potatoes

Carrot-Egg Potato Basket

- 2 tbsps refrigerated shredded hash brown potatoes
- 2 tbsps shredded carrot

Zucchini-Herb-Egg Potato Basket

- 2 tbsps of refrigerated shredded hash brown potatoes
- 2 tbsps of shredded zucchini, squeezed dry with clean

dish towel or paper towels

- 1 tsp of fresh flat-leaf parsley chopped
- 1/2 tsp of fresh chives chopped

Beet-Egg Potato Basket

- 2 tbsps of refrigerated shredded hash brown potatoes
- 2 tbsps of red beet peeled, shredded

You need two eggs for each recipe above.

Instructions

Using cooking oil, spray each muffin cup.

Mix the ingredients mentioned above in separate bowls for each egg basket form you're creating, omitting the eggs.

Divide that recipe in half, then spoon half of one half into one muffin cup as well as the other half into another muffin cup. Continue this process with each egg basket recipe you're creating.

Press the mixture lightly into the bottom & up the sides of each muffin cup, slightly above the rim (baskets shrink when baking).

Preheat oven to 350°F and bake for 30 minutes.

Remove the baskets from the oven, then crack one big

egg into each.

Return the muffin tin to the oven for another 12 to 15 minutes or until the eggs are cooked to your taste.

To taste, season with salt & pepper.

10. Gluten-Free Pancakes of Blueberry Banana

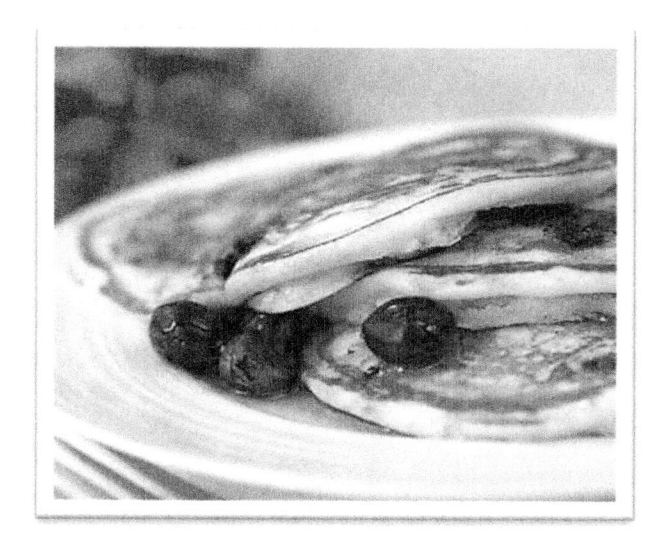

Prep time + Cook time: 10 minutes

Servings: 2

Ingredients

- 1 and 1/2 of ripe bananas
- Two eggs
- 1/8 tsp of baking powder
- 1/2 cup of fresh blueberries

- for serving, butter & maple syrup (optional)

Instructions

In a bowl, mash the peeled bananas with the fork or potato masher, making them mildly lumpy.

Whisk the eggs in a separate bowl before the yolks are split up and mixed with the egg whites.

Mix the bananas, eggs, and baking powder in a large mixing bowl.

Heat up a skillet (or saute pan) to medium heat when the baking powder is activating.

Using cooking spray, spray the heated griddle and add 2 tbsps of batter onto it.

Place a few blueberries in the batter as several tiny bubbles emerge on top of the pancake and flip to cook its other side.

Serve directly with a sprinkling of butter and a glaze of maple syrup.

11. Rhubarb Walnut Muffins

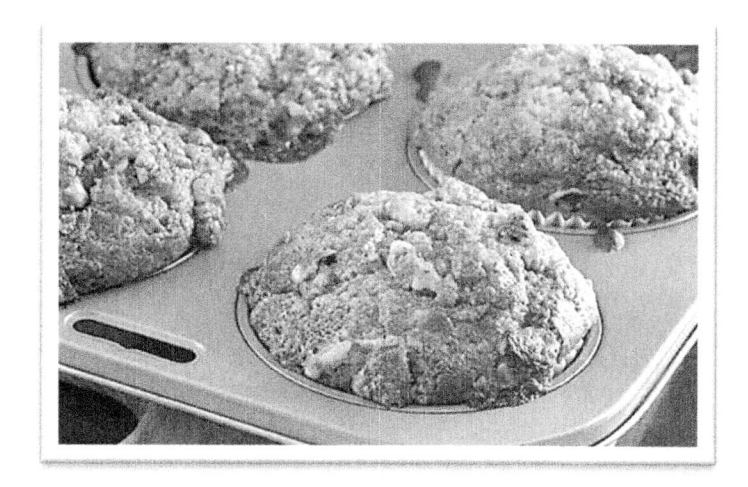

Though frozen rhubarb is available year-round, spring is the best time to pick fresh rhubarb from your greenhouse. Instead of the traditional strawberry/rhubarb muffin, try these Rhubarb Walnut Muffins.

Prep time + Cook time: 10 minutes

Servings: 2

Ingredients

For Muffins

- 1 1/2 cups of all-purpose flour (gluten-free is better)
- 3/4 cup of brown sugar
- 1/2 tsp of baking soda
- 1/2 tsp of salt

- 1/3 cup of vegetable oil
- One egg large size
- 1/2 cup of buttermilk
- 1 tsp of vanilla extract pure
- 1 cup of fresh rhubarb finely chopped (substitute frozen rhubarb which has been thawed & well-drained)
- 1/2 cup of walnuts chopped

For Topping

- 1/2 cup of brown sugar
- 1/4 cup of walnuts chopped
- 1/2 tsp of cinnamon

Instructions

Preheat the oven to 325 degrees Fahrenheit. Paper liners can be used to cover muffin tins.

Combine the flour, baking soda, brown sugar, and salt in a mixing bowl.

Combine the egg, vegetable oil, buttermilk, and vanilla in a separate bowl.

To avoid tough and heavy muffins, add the wet

ingredients to dry ingredients and blend only until mixed.

Combine the rhubarb and walnuts in a mixing bowl.

Spoon batter into muffin tins lined with paper liners to just below the tip of the paper liners.

To make the icing, mix all of the ingredients and brush on top of the muffins.

Bake for 20 - 25 minutes, or when a cake tester inserted in the middle comes out clean, and the tops are well browned.

6.2 Liver Friendly Appetizers, Soups and Salads

1. Easy Detox Quinoa Salad

Prep Time + Cook time: 5 minutes

Servings: 2

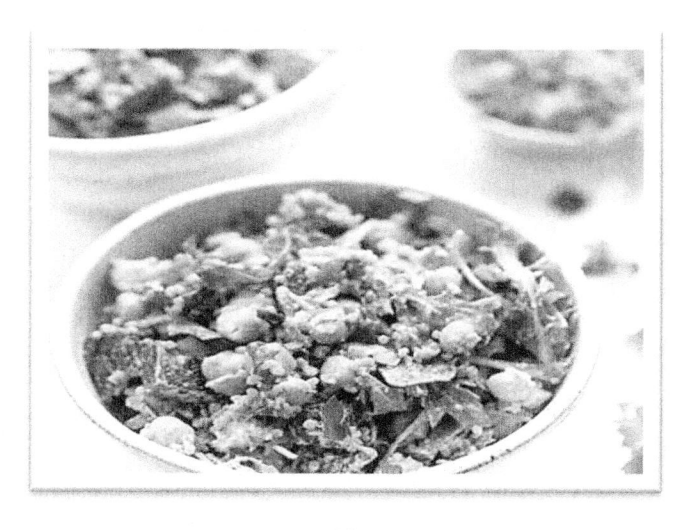

Ingredients

- 4 cups of arugula
- 1 cup of quinoa cooked
- 1 cup of cooked beets, diced, preferably organic
- 1 15 oz. can of drained and rinsed chickpeas

For Dressing:

- Juice of 1 Fresh lemon
- 2 tbsps of tahini
- 1 tbsps of coarse mustard
- One grated clove garlic
- 1 tbsp of water (if required)
- Salt & pepper for taste

Instructions

Mix all salad ingredients in a big mixing bowl.

Combine the vinaigrette ingredients in a mixing bowl. Toss the salad until it is well mixed.

Serve instantly or chill for 30 minutes (optional).

2. Detox Turmeric Lentil Soup

Prep Time + Cook time: 50 minutes

Servings: 6

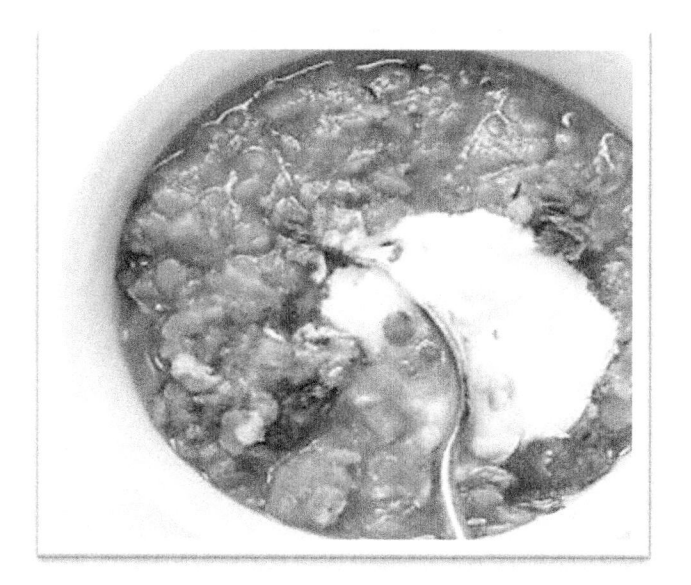

Ingredients

- 1 tbsp of avocado oil
- 1 cup of chopped onion
- 1 cup of chopped celery
- 1 cup of chopped potato or turnip
- 2 1/2 cups of sweet potato chopped
- Two garlic cloves minced
- 1 tsp of sea salt

- 1 tsp of black pepper
- 2 tsps of dried thyme
- 1 cup of brown or green lentils
- 1 cup of red lentils
- 2 tbsp of turmeric
- 1 tsp of ginger
- 1 tsp of cumin
- 4 cups of vegetable broth
- 2 cups of water
- 1 cup of almond milk
- 1 cup of spinach
- 1 cup of fresh herbs
- 1 tsp of lemon juice
- 1/2 tsp flakes of red pepper

Instructions

In a Dutch oven or large stockpot, heat the oil. Sauté the potatoes, celery, turnip, onion, and garlic for around 5 minutes, or until softened slightly. Cook for about 2 minutes, seasoning with salt, pepper, and thyme.

Sauté the turmeric, ginger, lentils and cumin for 1–2

minutes before adding the broth & water. Get the soup to just a boil, then reduce to low heat and cover for 30 minutes.

Remove from the heat and mix in the almond milk, herbs, spinach, lemon juice, and pepper flakes until the spinach is wilted. Serve immediately!

3. Detox Green Smoothie

Prep time + Cook time: 5 mints

Servings: 2

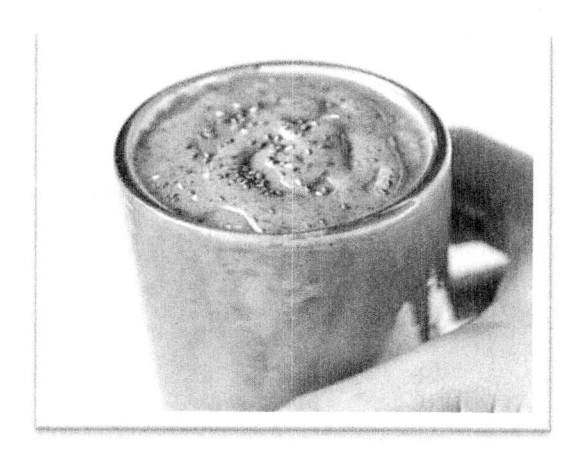

Ingredients

- 4 cups of greens (spinach, kale, etc.)
- 1 cup of chopped cucumber
- 1/2 cup of frozen cauliflower rice
- 1/4 cup of frozen raspberries

- One frozen banana
- 1/2 avocado
- 1 tbsp of chia seeds
- 1 tbsp of flaxseed meal
- 1 tbsp of almond butter
- 1" fresh ginger piece
- Juice of 1/2 lemon
- 1 cup of coconut water
- 1 cup of water (or use almond milk)

Instructions

Blend all together in a high-powered blender until smooth. Pour into a bowl, cover with toppings (if desired), and enjoy!

4. Maca Latte, Vegan & Caffeine-Free

Prep time + Cook time: 5 mints

Servings: 2

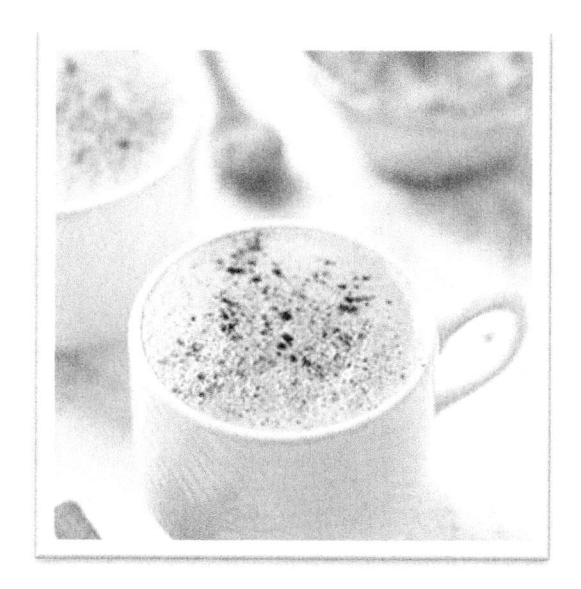

Ingredients

- 2 tsp of maca powder gelatinized
- 1 tsp of Chaga mushroom powder
- 1 tsp of ground cinnamon
- Monk fruit extract for Sprinkle
- 1 tbsp of MCT oil
- 1/2 cup of almond milk unsweetened
- 20 oz. of hot water

Instructions

In a blender, combine both of the ingredients. Blend on high until the mixture is creamy.

Divide the mixture equally between the two mugs. Topping each latte with a dollop of foam and a sprinkle of maca.

5. Liver Cleanse Soup

Prep time + Cook time: 75 mints

Servings: 4

Ingredients

- 3 cups of filtered or purified water
- 1 cup of broth organic vegetable
- Two peeled and diced organic beets
- Two sliced organic carrots
- 2 cups of chopped organic broccoli
- Ten cloves of freshly crushed organic garlic
- One diced organic onion
- 1/2 freshly squeezed organic lemon
- Two bay leaves organic
- 1/2 tsp of Himalayan pink salt

- 1/2 tsp of organic ground turmeric
- 1/2 tsp of organic dried oregano
- 1/2 tsp of ground black pepper organic

Instructions

To prepare the veggies:

Depending on your choice, cut/slice/dice the beets, broccoli, onions, and carrots to the desired amount.

To prepare the soup:

In a medium-sized pot, mix all of the soup's ingredients and bring to a boil.

Reduce the heat to low and simmer for around 1 hour, just until the vegetables are tender.

If necessary, add more water or veggie broth, and change seasonings to taste.

6. Creamy Vegetable Minestrone Soup

Prep time + Cook time: 30 mints

Servings: 4

Ingredients

- 1 cup of diced organic onion
- Three diced organic carrots

- Two diced organic Roma tomatoes
- One stalk diced organic celery
- Two freshly crushed cloves of organic garlic
- 2-3 tsp red pepper flakes organic
- 2 tsp of avocado oil 100% pure
- 1/2 tsp of pink salt Himalayan

For add-ins:

- 4 cups of vegetable broth organic
- 1 can (15-ounce can drained) of organic cannellini beans
- 1 can (13.5-ounce can) of full-fat coconut milk organic

For vegetable add-ins:

- 2 cups of chopped organic spinach
- 2 tbsps of chopped organic fresh parsley

Instructions

Prep the veggies:

Prepare the vegetables by dicing the onions, peppers, celery, and carrots and cutting the spinach and parsley.

Prepare the veggie saute':

In a saucepan or large pot, mix all of the ingredients for veggie saute' and cook over medium/high heat for 2 to 3 mints, or till the onions are tender.

Prepare the soup:

Simmer uncovered on low heat for 10-15 minutes with the cannellini beans, vegetable broth, and whole can of coconut milk.

Stir in the chopped spinach & parsley until it is well mixed and the spinach has wilted somewhat.

Season to taste and change seasonings as required.

Refrigerate any leftovers in an airtight BPA-free bag.

7. Creamy Kale and Red Lentil Soup

Prep time + Cook time: 40 mints

Servings: 4

Ingredients

For the soup:

- 1 1/2 cups of uncooked organic red lentils
- 2 cups of organic diced tomatoes
- 3 cups of organic vegetable broth
- 1/2 diced organic onion

- 2 tbsps of tomato sauce organic
- 1 1/2 tsps of organic ground cumin
- 1 tsp of pink salt Himalayan
- 1-2 pinches cayenne pepper organic

For add-ins:

- 1 cup of (destemmed, chopped) organic kale
- One can (13.5-ounce can) full-fat coconut milk organic

Instructions

Prepare the vegetables as follows: De-stem the kale, then chop into small strips; dice the onions and tomatoes.

In a medium-sized pot, mix all of the soup's ingredients, stir well, and then bring to a boil.

Reduce to a low/medium heat setting, cover, then cook for 25-30 minutes, or until lentils are tender. Stir periodically to avoid burning and, if necessary, apply a little more veggie broth.

Remove the lentils from the heat and stir in the chopped kale and the whole can of coconut milk.

To make sure it is well combined, give it a good stir. Seasonings may be tweaked to taste.

Have fun!

8. Asian Quinoa Power Salad

Prep Time + Cook time: 10 minutes

Servings: 4

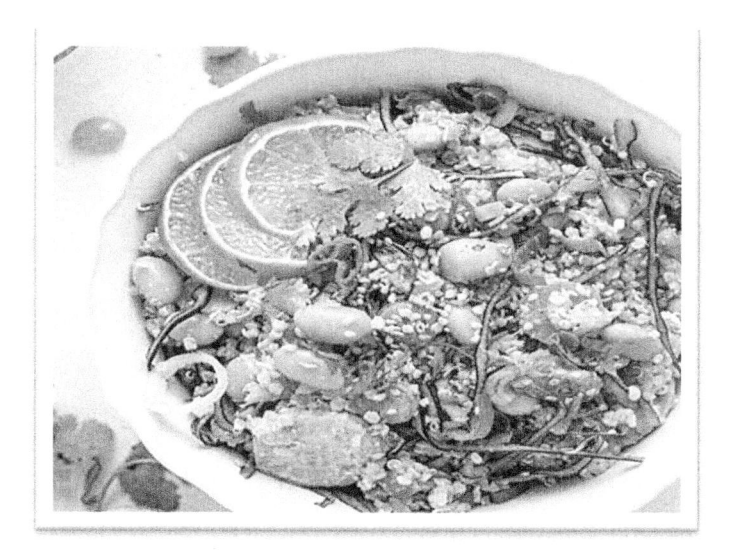

Ingredients

- 3 cups of cooked quinoa
- 1 cup of frozen-thawed edamame
- 1 cup of carrots thinly sliced
- 1 cup of finely chopped kale shredded red cabbage
- 1/2 cup of green onions thinly sliced
- 1/2 cup of chopped kimchi

- 1/3 cup of cilantro
- 1 Ginger-Miso Dressing batch

Instructions

In a big mixing bowl, mix all of the salad ingredients. Toss the salad with the dressing to combine it. Serve immediately.

9. Avocado with Cucumber Quinoa Salad

Prep time + Cook time: 10 mints

Servings: 4

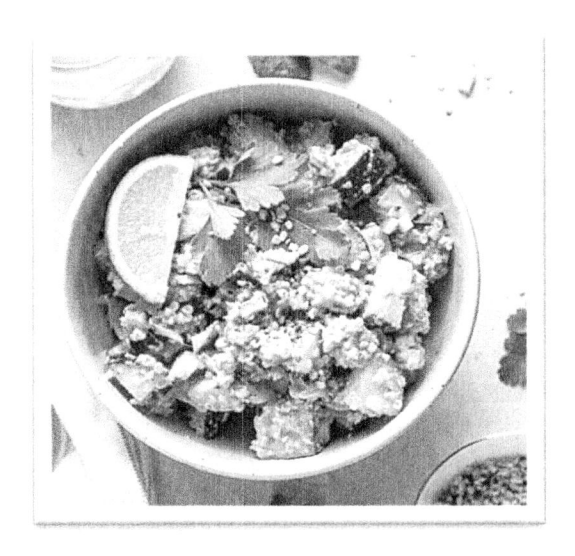

Ingredients

- 1 cucumber large size
- 1 avocado large size

- 1 cup of cooked quinoa
- 1/2 cup of red onion diced
- 1/2 - 3/4 dressing batch
- For garnish Hemp seeds (optional)

For Dressing:

- 1/3 cup of water
- 1/4 cup of raw cashews
- 1/4 cup of parsley
- 1/4 cup of cilantro
- 1/4 cup of spinach
- 2 scallions
- 1 lime for Juice
- 2 tsps of soy sauce
- Salt & pepper

Instructions

Remove the pit from the avocado and cut it in half. Scoop into a big mixing bowl and cut into bite-sized portions.

Cucumbers can be sliced lengthwise down the center. Then split it into three long, equal strips. The cucumber can then be chopped into cubes and added to the mixing cup.

Place aside the quinoa and onion.

In a high-powered blender, combine the water, cashews, herbs, spinach, lime juice, scallions and soy sauce. Blend on high speed until the mixture is thick and fluffy. Season with salt & pepper to taste, if necessary.

Toss around half to three-quarters of the dressing into the mixing bowl to blend. If you like to incorporate more dressing, go ahead and do so!

Serve with hemp seeds sprinkled on top.

10. Tomato Detox Soup

Prep time + Cook time: 65 mints

Servings: 4

Ingredients

- 1 pint of grape tomatoes
- 1 tbsp of olive oil grape-seed
- 1 tbsp of chopped ginger
- 1/2 cup of Vidalia onion chopped
- 3 cloves minced garlic 2 tbsp or garlic paste
- 2 cans of fire-roasted diced tomatoes (14.5 ounces)

- 1- quart of vegetable stock
- Fresh Basil about a handful
- Salt & black pepper
- Garnish: Pepitas

Instructions

Preheat the oven to 300 degrees Fahrenheit.

Roast the tomatoes for 35 minutes in a shallow baking dish or in aluminum foil (with top open). Enable them to stay in the oven for another 15 minutes after turning it off. If you're short on time, they will stay there before they cool off. If you like, you can do this ahead of time.) When you're about to create the soup, combine all of the ingredients in a large mixing bowl. In a medium pot, heat the oil and saute the onions & ginger for a few minutes. Add the garlic and roasted tomatoes, then continue to saute for a few minutes more. If desired, press down the tomatoes by the spoon or use potato masher to "pop" them.

Season with salt and pepper and bring to a boil with the canned tomatoes and vegetable reserve.

Simmer for 10 minutes, then add the basil and season again until you have the flavor you like.

Choose if you like the soup to be pureed or chunky. Using

an immersion blender or a regular blender. Soup can be pureed.

Enjoy it hot, cold, or room temperature. Enjoy! Garnish with a pinch of pepitas, chives or scallions, and basil.

11. Liver Detox Soup

Prep time + Cook time: 40 mints

Servings: 4

Ingredients

- 4 cups of water
- 3 cubes of vegetable stock
- 2 cups of beets
- 2 cups of carrot
- 2 cups of cauliflower
- 2 cloves of garlic
- 1 medium-size onion
- ½ cup of canned artichoke
- 1 tsp of olive oil
- ¼ tsp of salt
- ¼ tsp of pepper

Instructions

In a large pot, mix 4 cups water and 3 cubes vegetable stock. Get the water to boil in a large pot.

Beets, carrots, and cauliflower should be diced into 1-inch pieces and added to a pot of boiling water for vegetable stock. The cooking time is 30 minutes. Keep the soup covered and on a low boil to prevent so much water from escaping; otherwise, you may need extra water at the end.

Garlic, onion, and artichoke can both be finely diced. Cook for 10 minutes in a skillet of olive oil over medium heat. Salt and pepper to taste.

Add the sauteed vegetables to the pot after the beet, carrot, and cauliflower have finished frying. Using an immersion blender, mix all of the veggies into a creamy soup.

12. Detox Cabbage Soup

Prep time + Cook time: 20

Servings: 2-3

Ingredients

- 1 tbsp of ghee or coconut oil (or any choice of healthy Fat)
- 1/2 sliced thinly small cabbage

- 3 stalks of chopped celery
- 1/2 tsp of salt
- 2 cloves minced garlic
- 1/2–1 tsp of fresh ginger grated
- 2 and 1/2 cups good quality broth (veggie broth or bone broth)
- 1 cup shredded or chopped leftover chicken (use meat if you like)
- Cilantro (fresh) for garnish

Instructions

In a soup pot at medium-high heat, melt the Fat of your preference. Combine the cabbage, celery, and salt in a large mixing bowl. Cook, stirring regularly, for 3-4 minutes, or until the vegetables begin to soften. Cook for another minute after adding the garlic and ginger.

Add the broth and chicken to the pot and boil until the vegetables are tender.

Serve directly with fresh cilantro as a garnish. Keep leftovers for up to 2 days in an airtight glass jar.

13. Easy Detox Soup

Prep time + Cook time: 30 mints

Servings: 6

Ingredients

- 2 tbsps of olive oil (30 ml)
- 1 cup of peeled and chopped red onion
- 1 cup of chopped bell pepper
- 1 cup sliced celery
- 3 tbsps of minced or grated fresh ginger
- 4 minced garlic cloves
- 2 chicken breasts, boneless and skinless (about 1 lb.)
- 8 cups of chicken bone broth
- 1 cup of sliced carrots
- 1 tbsp of vinegar **apple cider**
- 1/4 tsp of **ground turmeric**
- ¼ tsp of **ground cumin**
- 1/4 tsp of cayenne pepper
- 1 cup of broccoli florets
- 1 cup of destemmed kale, torn in pieces

- Salt and freshly cracked black pepper for taste
- 1/4 cup of parsley chopped
- Thinly sliced chilies for serving

Instructions

Pressure Cooker

Set the pressure cooker at "sauté" and increase the setting to "more. When the pan is wet, add the olive oil. Then add the onions, peppers, celery, ginger, & garlic, then cook, often stirring, for 3-4 minutes, or until softened but not browned.

Mix together the fresh chicken breasts, broth, carrots, apple cider vinegar, cumin, turmeric, and cayenne pepper.

Cover the pressure release valve and secure the cover to the instant pot. Choose "High Pressure" and set the timer for 10 minutes.

As the timer goes off, click "cancel" and quickly release the pressure, ensuring the pressure valve is adjusted to vent.

Using two forks, shred the chicken from the pot.

Select "sauté" mode and increase the heat. In a large mixing bowl, add the shredded chicken, broccoli & kale.

Cook until broccoli is soft, around 6–8 minutes. If required, season with more salt & pepper.

If needed, garnish with parsley & thinly sliced chilies. Serve immediately.

Stovetop

Heat the olive oil in a large pot over medium-high heat. Then add the onions, peppers, celery, ginger & garlic then cook, stirring often, for 3-4 minutes, or until softened but not browned.

Mix together the fresh chicken breasts, carrots, apple cider vinegar, turmeric, cumin, broth and cayenne pepper.

Get the liquid to boil, then decrease to a low heat. Cover and cook for 20 to 25 minutes, or until the chicken is well cooked through and the vegetables are tender.

Using two forks, shred the chicken from the pot.

Return the shredded chicken to the pot, together with the broccoli and kale, and toss to blend. Cook until broccoli is soft, around 6–8 minutes. If required, season with more salt & pepper.

14. Crunchy Liver detox salad

Prep Time + Cook time: 20 mints

Servings: 2 people

Ingredients

- 1 clove of garlic
- 1 red onion small size
- 1 cup of red cabbage
- 1 ginger slice
- 1 cup of cilantro
- Leaves sage few
- black radish small piece
- 1 cup of cooked cold quinoa
- 1 lemon
- 15 almonds
- pinch salt
- 1 tbsp of olive oil Cold-pressed

Instructions

To begin, mince the garlic and place it in a salad bowl.

Place the red cabbage, onion, and shredded red

cabbage in a mixing bowl and stir to mix.

You have the choice of chopping the cilantro or only using the leaves. Place it in a bowl with sage leaves and put it aside.

Cut black radish into very thin slices and combine with cilantro.

If you like, you can chop your almonds or leave them whole.

To get the juice from your lemon, squeeze it. If your lemon is organic, dice any lemon skin if needed.

Put all into the bowl to make the crunchy Liver detox salad. Gently combine and serve.

You can now eat the salad. Good relaxation.

15. An Extremely Simple Salad

Prep time + Cook time: 15 mints

Servings: 1

Ingredients

Salad

- 2 large handfuls of rocket arugula
- 1 small beetroot

- 1/2 avocado
- 2 radishes
- 1 tbsp of parsley, chopped
- 1 tbsp of walnuts, chopped

Dressing

- 1 cup of walnut oil (250 ml)
- 1 tsp of apple cider vinegar
- 2 tsp of honey
- juice of ½ lemon
- ¼ cup of washed and chopped fresh parsley
- 1 garlic clove
- Salt and pepper, for taste

Instruction

Salad:

Everything produce should be thoroughly washed.

Remove the ends of the beets and peel them. Greens can be saved for juicing.

Place arugula in a bowl after drying it with paper towels.

Using a mandolin, slice beets & radishes into salad

Chop walnuts to your liking.

Parsley can be chopped.

Round the avocado in half all the way through and rotate to divide the halves. Remove the pit and spoon out the flesh before slicing. Save the pit from the other half of the avocado for further use (add lemon to prevent browning).

Starting with the arugula, layer the salad, finishing with the parsley.

Dressing:

In a mixer, add walnut oil, honey, and apple cider vinegar. Start with 1 tsp honey and 1 tsp apple cider vinegar, then apply more of one or both to taste.

Squeeze the lemon into the mixer and combine it with the other ingredients.

Parsley should be washed and chopped before being added to a blender and mixed.

To cut the peel from the garlic, smash it with a spoon and place it in a blender with the ingredients' rest.

Add salt and pepper to the blender and mix on low to medium until smooth, or whisk rapidly in a bowl until smooth.

Pour 1-2 tbsps of dressing over salad, then keep the rest refrigerated in an airtight container. It lasts for seven days in the fridge.

16. Detox Salad with Ginger-Lemon Dressing

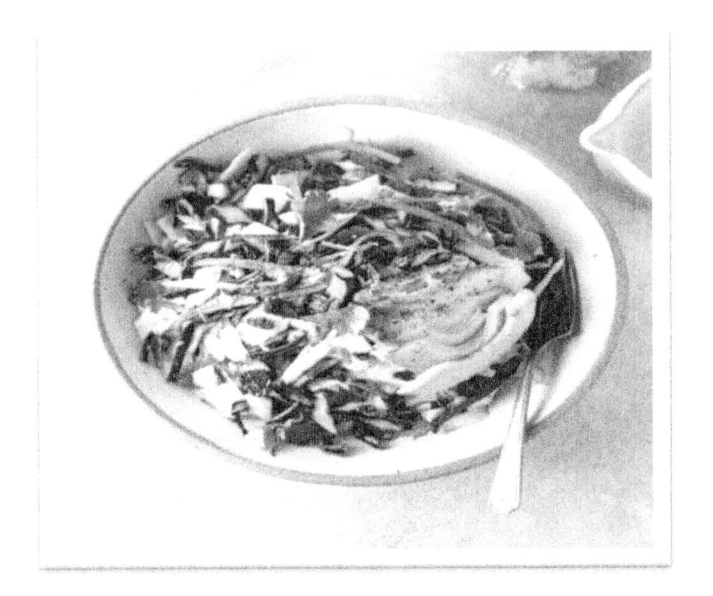

Prep time + Cook time: 10 mints

Servings: 2

Ingredients

Ginger Lemon Dressing

- 3/4 cup of freshly squeezed lemon juice
- 1/2 cup of extra-virgin olive oil
- 1 clove of garlic

- 1 to 1 1/2-inch knob fresh ginger, for taste
- 2 tbsps of raw honey

Salad

- 4 cups of shredded cabbage (purple, green, or both)
- A handful of roughly chopped fresh flat-leaf parsley
- One large shredded carrot
- 2 tbsps raisins
- 1/2 sliced avocado

Instructions

To make the dressing, mix all of the materials in a blender until smooth, beginning with only 1-inch fresh ginger. If needed, add more ginger for taste and set aside.

To make the salad, mix the cabbage, carrots, & parsley in a large mixing bowl, then add the sliced avocado & raisins on top.

Before eating, whipped topping 3 to 4 tsps of the lemon-ginger seasoning over the assembled salad and set aside for 5 to 10 minutes to marinate. Refrigerate any remaining dressing in an airtight jar for up to a week.

17. Seafood Salad

Prep time + Cook time: 15 mints

Servings: 2

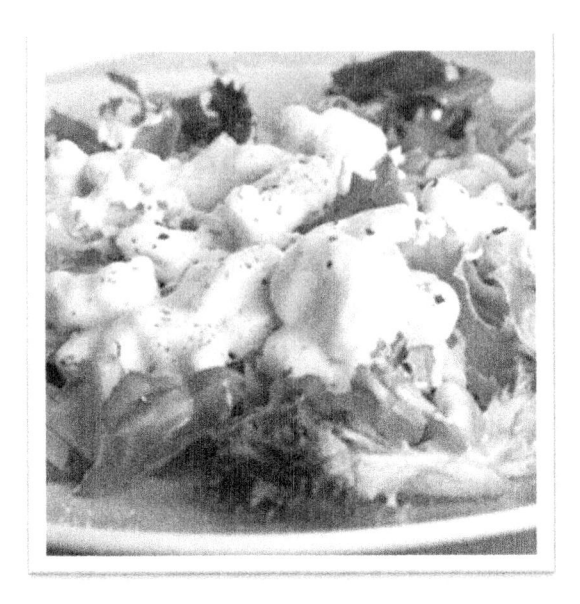

Ingredients

- 2 tbsps of light mayonnaise
- 1/2 juice from lemon
- 1 cup (about 1/3 pound) cooked crabmeat, shredded, or imitation crabmeat,
- 1 cup of cooked bay shrimp (about 1/3 pound)
- 1/3 cup of fat-free or light sour cream
- 1/2 cup of chopped celery

- 6 cups of chopped Romaine, or spinach or green leaf lettuce
- 1/4 tsp of salt, optional
- 2 tbsps of sliced black olives
- 1/4 tsp of pepper freshly ground, add more for taste
- 1 chopped green onion

Instructions

In a medium mixing bowl, combine light mayonnaise, sour cream, and lemon juice.

Add the crab, shrimp, celery, salt, olives, pepper and green onions and stir to blend. Allow at least 1 hour for chilling.

Each helping of seafood salad should be served on a bed of 2 cups of lettuce greens.

18. Low-Carb Taco

Prep Time + Cook Time: 30 min

Servings: 5

Ingredients

- 1 pound of lean ground beef (84% to 90% lean)
- 8 white and green parts separated green onions,

chopped,

- 1 tbsp of chili powder
- 1 head chopped romaine lettuce
- 1 diced avocado
- 1 medium chopped tomato
- 1 4-ounce can olives sliced
- 1 1/2 cups of grated fat-free cheese, Monterey Jack, or a combination, Cheddar
- 1/2 cup of salsa
- 1/2 cup of plain yogurt or fat-free Greek

Instructions

In a skillet, cook the beef with chili powder, the white portion of the onions, salt and pepper. If you want the beef warm before you add it to the salad, cover the pan; if you want it chilled, put it in the refrigerator before you're going to assemble the salad.

Mix the lettuce, avocado, tomato, olives and green onion, if using, in a large salad bowl. Toss in the meat and cheese with a gentle hand. Place in serving bowls that share at the table and top with dollops of yogurt & salsa.

Appetizers

1. Baked Zucchini Fries

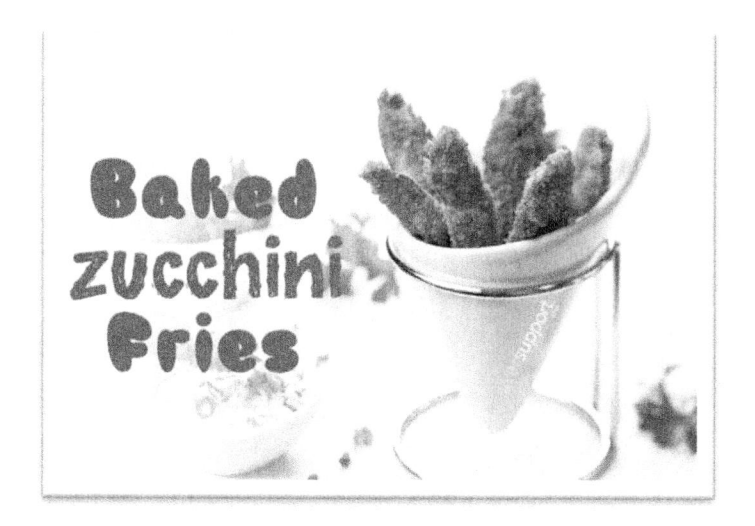

Prep Time + Cook Time: 25 mints

Servings: 4-6

Ingredients

- 2 to 3 med. Size zucchini cut into fries
- 1/4 tsp of salt
- 1/4 cup of flour
- 1/4 tsp of garlic powder
- 1/2 cup of milk (any kind you like)
- 1/4 cup of Vegan Parmesan cheese
- 1 cup of Panko breadcrumbs

Instructions

Preheat the oven to 425 degrees Fahrenheit.

Using parchment paper, line a baking sheet.

Mix the flour, salt, garlic powder, and Vegan Parmesan Cheese in a shallow bowl or pie plate.

Pour the milk into a separate bowl.

Bread crumbs should be placed in a bowl or pie plate.

Place the zucchini on the lined baking sheet, leaving space for each slice, after dipping it in the flour mixture, and the milk, then finally the breadcrumbs.

Bake for 20 minutes, or until crispiness is required. NOTE: You should finish in the broiler around 2 minutes for extra crispiness.

Serve with marinara sauce, dairy-free ranch dressing, or tzatziki sauce.

2. Fresh Corn Salsa

Prep Time + Cook Time: 18 Mints

Servings: 8

Ingredients

- 3 ears of shucked fresh corn on the cob

- 1/4 cup of minced red onion
- 2 tsp of finely diced jalapeños (seeds & membranes removed)
- 1/4 cup of finely chopped fresh cilantro
- 1/2 tsp sea salt
- Juice from one lime

Instructions

Preheat the grill to medium.

On the preheated grill, cook the shucked corn rotating periodically, for around 10 minutes, or until the corn is soft and specks of black develop on the kernels. Set aside until completely cool.

Remove the corn kernels from the cob and place them in a dish.

Stir in the remaining ingredients until it is well mixed.

3. Healthy Nachos (grain, dairy-free, soy)

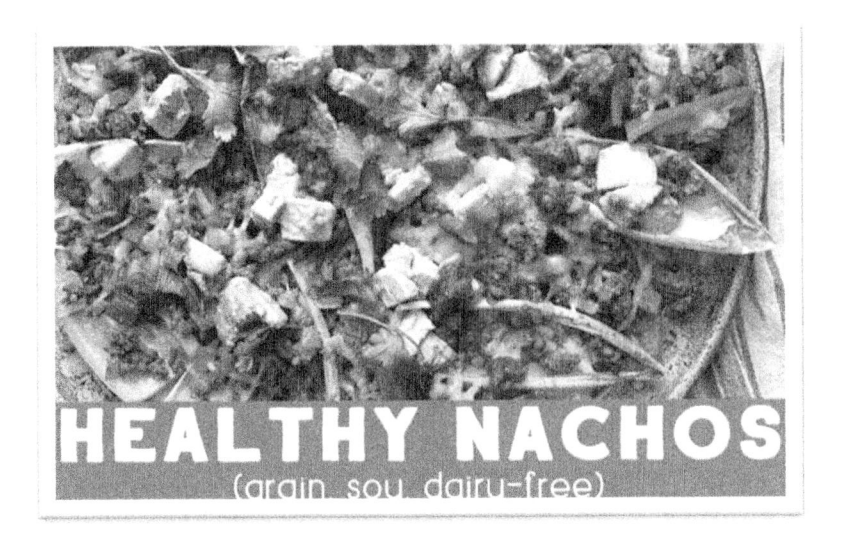

Ingredients

Tacos

- 2 Tbsp of olive oil
- 1 medium-small diced yellow onion
- 1 small diced medium zucchini
- Taco seasoning (your favorite)
- 7-8 cut in half cherry tomatoes
- 2 tsp of minced garlic
- 1 lime
- 10 bell peppers mini sweet stem removed, scooped out, cut in half

- 1 lb. of ground turkey
- 10 leaves of endive
- 1 cup of vegan regular mozzarella cheese (if preferred)
- 1 small peeled avocado, pit removed, diced
- cilantro leaves a small handful
- Pepper to taste
- Salt to taste
- Salsa (your favorite brand)

Taco Seasoning

- 1 Tbsp of ground cumin
- 1 Tbsp of smoked paprika ground
- 1 Tbsp of garlic powder
- 1 tsp of ground allspice
- 1/4 tsp of ground cinnamon

Instructions

Mix the olive oil, zucchini, taco seasoning, garlic, onion, and cherry tomatoes in a cast iron pan. Season with salt & pepper and cook until the onion is translucent and the tomatoes have broken down around 10 minutes.

If necessary, add a few tbsps of water to free the fond from the plate.

Cook the ground turkey on moderately low heat until there is no longer moisture in the pan.

Place the peppers and endive in a single layer on a pizza pan. Add 1/2 cup vegan cheese on top.

Top the peppers and endive with the vegetables and meat mixture and the remaining cheese. Broil for 1-2 minutes, or until the cheese is only melted.

In a mixing bowl, mix the avocado and a splash of juice from the lime. Season to taste with salt and toss all around. Add a couple of spoonful of your salsa and cilantro leaves to the top of the nachos. If desired, squeeze even more lime juice evenly over the nachos.

4. Cashew-Less Queso Dip Vegan

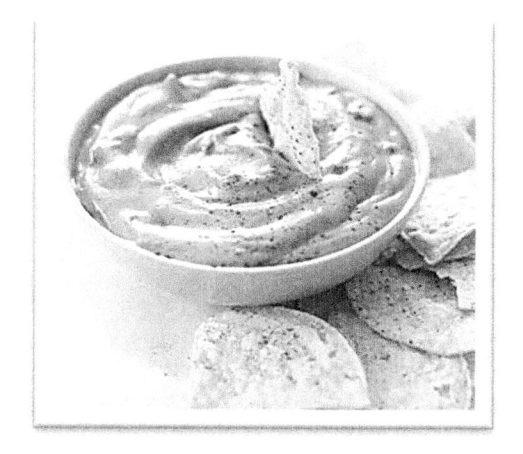

Prep time + Cook time: 45 mints

Servings: 6

Ingredients

- 8-9 sliced 1/4-inch thick rounds of eggplant (half of a med. eggplant)
- Sea salt
- Olive oil
- 1.5-2 cups of original almond milk unsweetened
- 2-3 tbsp of nutritional yeast
- 1 tsp of cumin
- 1/4 tsp of fresh garlic finely minced
- 1 tsp of chili powder

- 1/4 cup of slightly drained chunky salsa
- 2 tsp of cornstarch

Instructions

Slice the eggplant into thin rounds that are somewhat less than 1/2 inch thick (but not yet 1/4 inch). Then, to help draw away more of the moisture and bitterness, sprinkle all sides of the meat with a little sea salt and place in a colander. Allow for 10-15 minutes of resting time. After that, rinse with cold water and dry absolutely between two clean towels.

Preheat the oven to high broil, then place an oven rack close to the end. Arrange the dry eggplant rounds on a baking tray that has been gently coated with nonstick spray and drizzled with olive oil on both sides. Using a pinch of salt, season to taste.

Broil for 4-5 minutes on either side on warm, keeping an eye on them, so they don't burn. To ensure even cooking, flip halfway through. Remove the eggplant from the oven until it is tender & both sides have a golden brown hue and cover it loosely in foil to steam.

Unwrap and remove the eggplant skin after a few minutes. It should be easy to remove. It will be almost 1 cup if you pack roasted eggplant into a one-cup measuring cup.

Blend eggplant, almond milk (start with the smallest amount), nutritional yeast (start with the smallest amount), minced garlic, chili powder, cumin, and cornstarch in a high-powered blender until smooth and fluffy. Season to taste and change seasonings if required. Or increased the amount of nutritional yeast and applied a pinch of sea salt. Add more almond milk to thin it out.

Heat in a small saucepan over medium to medium-high heat, occasionally stirring, until slightly thickened and bubbly, around 5 minutes. The heavier it becomes, the longer you go.

NOTE: If it isn't thick enough, make a cornstarch slurry by combining an extra 1 tsp cornstarch, a little almond milk, and 2-3 Tbsps of the cheese mixture in a small bowl Return to the pot after stirring to mix. It should thicken up nicely as a result of this.

Remove from heat until hot and thickened, then stir in DRAINED Rote or salsa I. If you add the solvent in, it will make the mixture runny. Pour into a dish and season with smoked paprika and hot sauce, if desired.

Serve with chips, vegetables or crackers as a side dish. Warm in a crockpot or, if you have one, over a tea light warmer. It fits great in the microwave.

NOTE: If you leave this dip out for a long time, it will lose its orange color. It doesn't change the taste, but it doesn't look appealing, so it's better to eat it right away!

Keep leftovers refrigerated and covered. In the fridge or a saucepan, it reheats well. It can hold for a few days, but it is better when it is new.

5. Vegan Cauliflower Wings

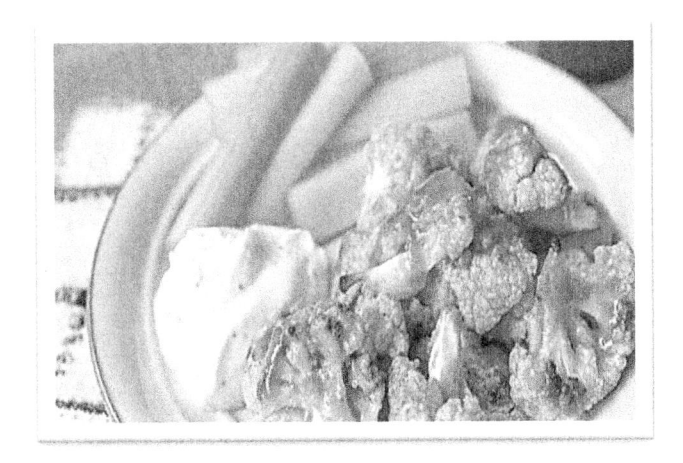

Prep time + Cook time: 60 mints

Serving: 6

Ingredients

For Wings

- 1 large (cut into florets) head of cauliflower

- 1/2 cup of water
- 1/2 cup of almond milk unsweetened
- 3/4 cup of all-purpose or rice flour
- 2 tsp of garlic powder
- 2 tsps of onion powder
- 1 tsp of cumin
- 1/4 tsp of ground pepper
- 1 tsp of paprika
- 1/4 tsp of sea salt

BBQ Sauce

- 1 tbsp of melted vegan butter
- Bottled sauce, your favorite!

Sauce Salt & Vinegar

- sea salt, for taste
- 1 tbsp of melted vegan butter
- 1 tbsp of water
- 3 tbsps of apple cider vinegar

Instructions

Preheat the oven to 450 degrees Fahrenheit.

Preheat oven to 350°F. Line baking sheets (two) with parchment paper.

In a large bowl, mix all of the Wing components.

Toss each cauliflower floret in the mixture and tap off any excess on the bowl's rim.

A place that dipped florets in such a single layer on the baking sheets that have been prepared.

Bake for 15 minutes before flipping and browning the other hand.

Cook for a further 10 minutes, or until golden brown.

In two different wide pots, prepare the sauce of choice (or both) when baking.

Remove the cauliflower florets from the oven and throw them in the sauce(s) to cover.

Place the florets in a single layer back onto the baking sheets. Sprinkle these cauliflower florets by sea salt if you're using the Salt & Vinegar sauce.

Bake for an additional 25 minutes, tossing the florets halfway round.

6. Cauliflower Crust Pizza

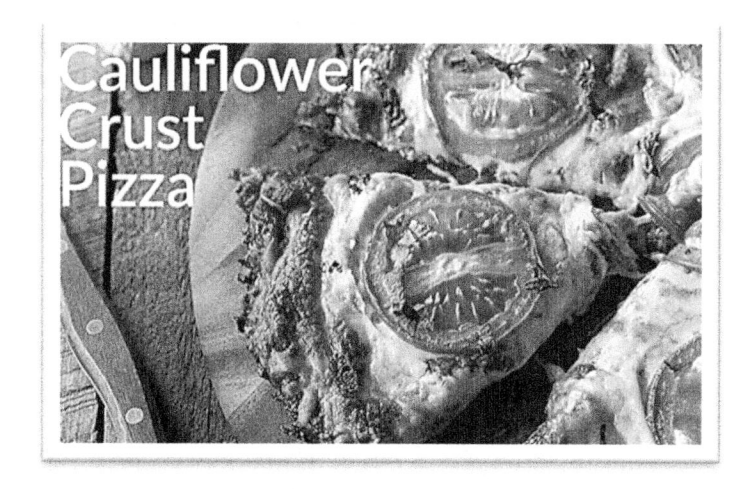

Prep time + Cook time: 45 mints

Servings: 6-8

Ingredients

- 1 cup of grated Parmesan
- 1 small chopped head cauliflower (about 6 cups)
- 1/2 tsp of Italian seasoning dried
- 1/2 tsp of kosher salt
- 1 minced clove of garlic
- black pepper freshly ground
- Olive oil
- 1 egg

- 1 1/2 cups of shredded mozzarella low-moisture
- 1/4 cup of freshly torn basil leaves
- 1 thinly sliced tomato (optional)
- 1/2 cup of marinara sauce

Instructions

Preheat the oven to 475 degrees F and place a baking sheet or pizza stone (upside down) in it.

In a food processor, pulse the cauliflower until it is finely ground.

To squeeze out enough liquid as necessary, pour the cauliflower over to a clean kitchen towel & twist both ends together.

Mix the cauliflower, Parmesan, garlic, Italian seasoning, salt, black pepper, and the egg in a large mixing bowl. If you pinch the mixture, it can stay together.

Use parchment paper to line the pizza peel or just a second upside-down baking sheet, then liberally spray with olive oil. On the parchment, spread the cauliflower paste into a 12-inch-wide shell. Place the parchment on the oven's baking sheet or preheated pizza stone. Bake for 15 minutes, or till the cauliflower crust becomes barely golden and thicker around the edges.

Remove the crust from oven, add half of the mozzarella on top, then layer the marinara sauce on top (to prevent the crust from drying out), then finish with the remaining mozzarella. Serve with tomato slices on top (optional). Transfer the pizza to the baking sheet or pizza stone and bake for 4 minutes, or until bubbly and browned in places.

Take the pizza out of the oven and sprinkle the basil on top. Cut into slices and serve.

7. Garden Hummus

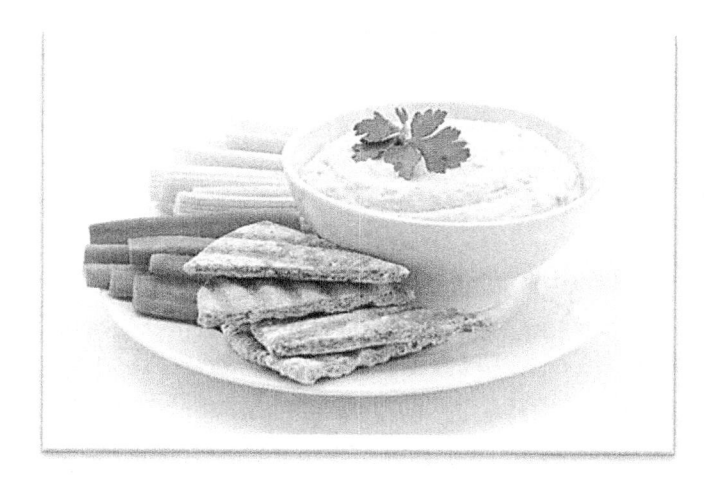

Prep time + Cook time: 60 mints

Servings: 4

Ingredients

- 1½ cups of garbanzo beans rinsed and soaked overnight

- 2 tbsps of olive oil
- 2 cloves of fresh garlic
- 1 jalapeno pepper, white flesh, and seeded removed to reduce the heat
- Freshly ground black pepper and salt for taste
- ¼ cup of distilled water
- tsp of cayenne pepper
- Juice of ½ lemon
- 1 tsp of paprika

Instructions

In a saucepan, simmer the beans. Cook for 60 minutes or until vegetables is soft. Then relax.

Jalapeno pepper & garlic cloves, roughly chopped.

Remove the stems from the parsley plants. Stems can be discarded.

In a food processor, blend the beans, vegetables, lemon juice, parsley, oil, cayenne, and paprika.

To achieve the perfect consistency, slowly add water to food processor when pulsing.

Season to taste with salt and pepper.

To serve, place in a bowl. Garnish with paprika and a few parsley leaves.

Dip with tortilla chips or a variety of fresh veggies.

8. Turkey Meatballs with Cranberry

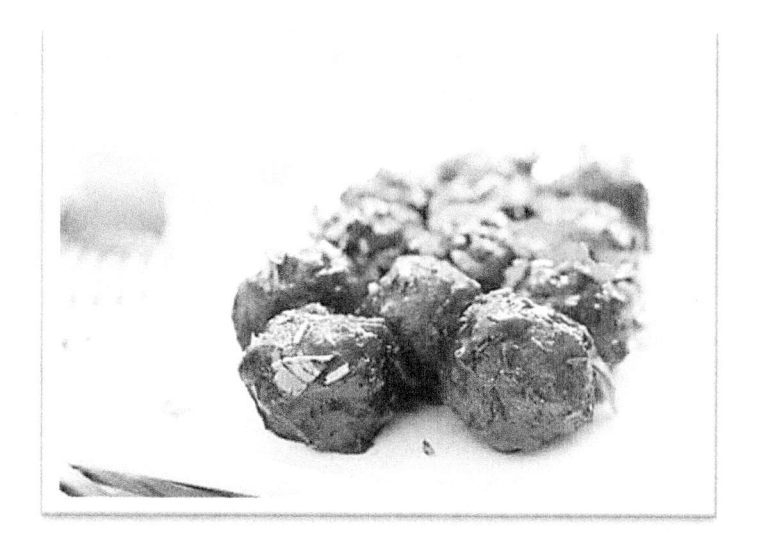

Prep time + Cook time: 45 mints

Servings: 4

Ingredients

- One large beaten egg
- 1¼ pounds of ground turkey
- ¼ tsp of poultry seasoning
- ½ tsp of garlic powder
- 1 tsp of onion powder

- 1 tsp of salt
- ½ tsp of black pepper
- ½ tsp of Worcestershire sauce
- 1 pinch of cayenne pepper
- ¼ cup of low-fat milk
- 1 7-ounce can of jellied cranberry sauce
- ½ cup of bread crumbs plain
- 1 tbsp of olive oil
- ½ cup of orange marmalade
- ½ cup of water
- Salt & pepper for taste

Instructions

In a large bowl, beat the egg.

Mix the turkey, poultry seasoning, onion powder, salt, garlic powder, black pepper, cayenne pepper (if desired), milk, Worcestershire sauce, and bread crumbs in the same mixing bowl. Mix the ingredients together with a spoon or your clean hands before they are just mixed.

Cover with plastic wrap and place in the refrigerator for 1 hour to make them set up more securely.

Remove one tbsp of the turkey mixture from the refrigerator and roll it into a ball. (Use a shallow cookie scoop or a tbsp scale to hold the balls the same size.)

In a pan, melt the olive oil over low heat.

Place that turkey meatballs in the skillet in a single sheet, making sure they don't touch. Through leaving enough space between the meatballs, you will guarantee that they brown rather than steam. You will need to brown the meatballs into batches depending on the scale of your skillet.

Brown the meatballs on both sides for about 3 minutes, rotating periodically.

Remove the skillet's meatballs before they begin to brown and position them on a clear baking sheet lined by paper towels to absorb any extra moisture or oils.

Add the cranberry sauce, marmalade, and water after all of the meatballs have been browned and extracted from the skillet. Gently stir the cranberry sauce & marmalade into the meatballs, removing some browned pieces off from bottom of the pan.

Bring the sauce to such a lively simmer, then cook for 3 minutes.

Toss the turkey meatballs back into the skillet.

Reduce the heat to medium-low and cook for another 5 minutes, or until the meatballs are not pink in the center and the glaze has decreased.

Periodically stir in the sauce and coat the turkey balls with it.

Season to taste with salt and pepper.

9. Guacamole

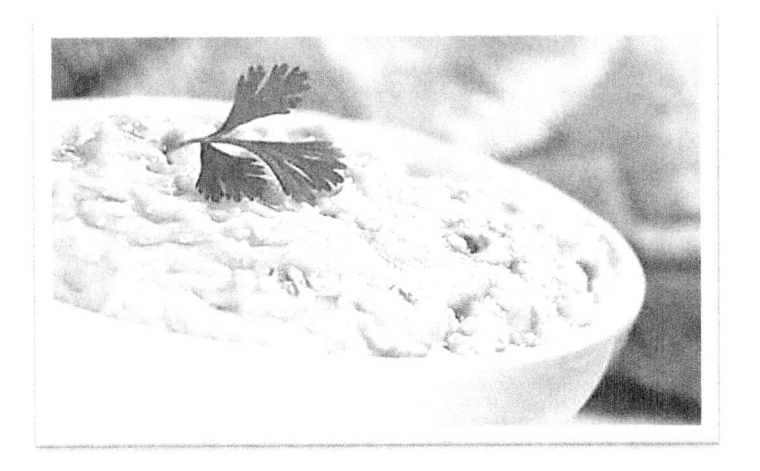

Prep time + Cook time: 15 mints

Servings: 2

Ingredients

- 3 avocados ripe
- 1 lime

- ½ cup of red onion small-diced (1 small onion)
- 1 pinch of ground cayenne pepper
- 1 tsp of salt
- 3 tbsps of fresh cilantro, chopped
- 3-4 minced garlic cloves
- 2 plum of tomatoes, diced and seed

Instructions

In a large bowl, cut the avocados in two, scrape the pits, and then scoop the flesh out from the pods. One pit can be set aside.

Cut the avocados in bowl with a sharp knife before desired quality is achieved. If you want a chunkier avocado, go ahead and do so.

Squeeze the lime juice into the bowl after cutting it in half (a reamer helps with that).

Mix in the salt, tomato, cilantro, onions, garlic, and cayenne pepper; don't break down the avocado into such a paste (unless that's your preference).

Serve immediately, or put the reserved pit in bowl (this will help keep the avocado from browning), cover the bowl by plastic wrap, so it touches the guacamole and refrigerate for up to 24 hours.

Serve with pita chips after removing the pit.

10. Pita Chips

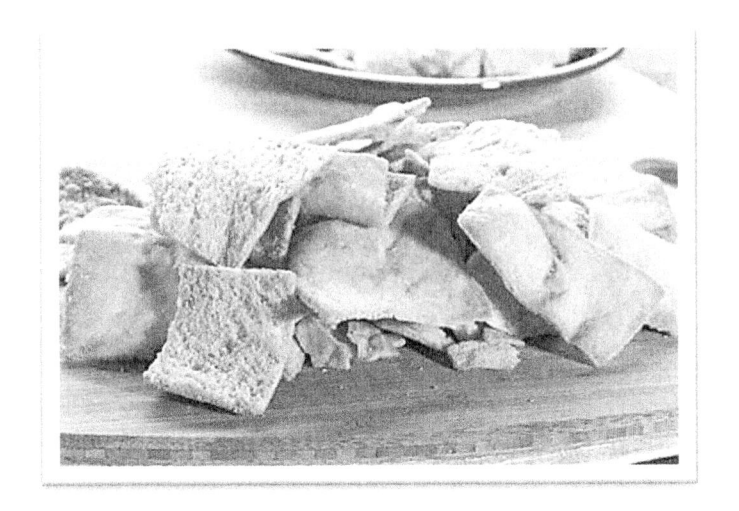

Prep time + Cook time: 13 mints

Servings: 2

Ingredients

- 2 tsps of olive oil
- 6 pitas whole wheat (without or with pocket)
- Chili powder
- Salt
- Garlic powder

Instructions

Preheat the oven to 400 degrees Fahrenheit.

Cut each pita in half, then into eight wedges, then arrange them on wide baking sheets, so they don't overlap.

Use an oil mister to gently mist the pitas with only enough olive oil to cause the spices to adhere (if you don't have an oil mister, brush the pitas with olive oil sparingly).

Garlic powder, chili powder, and salt can be lightly sprinkled on the pita wedges.

Preheat oven to 350°F and bake for 8 minutes, or until lightly golden.

Serve with hummus, Pico de Gallo, or a dip.

11. Pico de Gallo

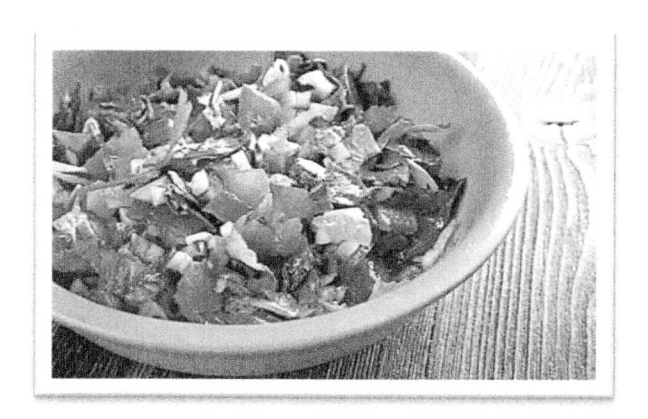

Prep time + Cook time: 15 mints

Servings: 2

Ingredients

- 1 large very finely diced, white or red onion
- 1½ cups of finely chopped fresh cilantro
- 10 vine tomatoes or 12 Roma tomatoes
- 3 finely chopped jalapenos with seeds and membranes removed
- ¼ tsp of salt
- 1 lime
- for serving Pita chips

Instructions

To begin, finely dice the onion and put it in a large bowl.

To make a tomato core, cut the tomato in half and remove the core. One by one, slice the tomatoes, so you have the equivalent quantity of diced tomato as onion.

Remove the stems from cilantro before preparing it. It's good if the small stems persist. Chop the cilantro finely.

Pick the seeds and membrane (which makes jalapenos spicy) by scraping them out by a spoon after cutting the jalapenos in half. The jalapeno can be cut into pieces and diced quite finely.

Toss the onions with the tomatoes, cilantro, & jalapeno.

Round the lime in half and pour half of the lime juice into the mixing cup (a reamer helps with that).

Stir in the salt until it is evenly mixed in the bowl.

If required, seasoning the Pico de Gallo with salt to taste. You will just want to add a little more lime juice from other half of the lime.

Serve with Tortillas or Pita Chips.

6.3 Lunch Recipes For Fatty Liver
1. Cannellini Bean Salad

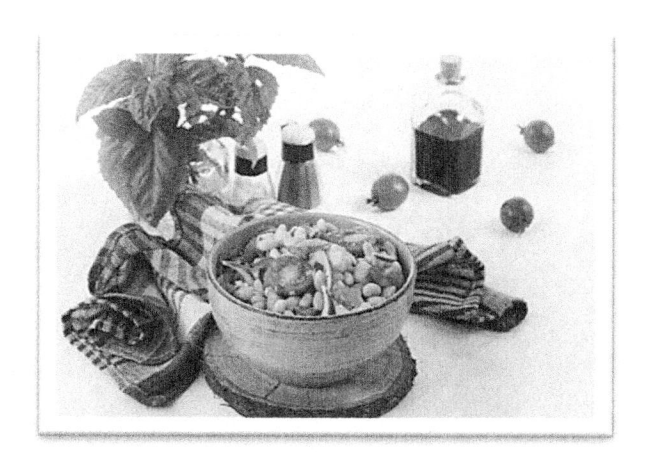

Prep time + Cook time: 5 minutes

Servings: 2

Ingredients

- 3 cups (600g) cannellini beans
- ⅜ cup (70g) halved cherry tomatoes
- ½ thinly sliced, red onion
- ½ tbsp. of red wine vinegar
- A small bunch of basil, torn

Instructions

Rinse, drain the beans, and blend them with the tomatoes, vinegar, and onion and in a mixing bowl.

Season with salt and pepper, then apply basil just before eating.

2. Carrot, Orange and Avocado Salad

Prep time + Cook time: 5 minutes

Servings: 2

Ingredients

- 1 orange
- sliced with a peeler and halved lengthways carrots
- ½ cups of arugula/ rocket
- 2 avocado, peeled and sliced, stoned
- 1 tbsp of olive oil

Instructions

Cut one of the oranges into segments and mix with the carrots, arugula, and avocado in a bowl. Mix the zest, orange juice, and oil in a mixing bowl. Season with salt and pepper.

3. Panzanella Salad

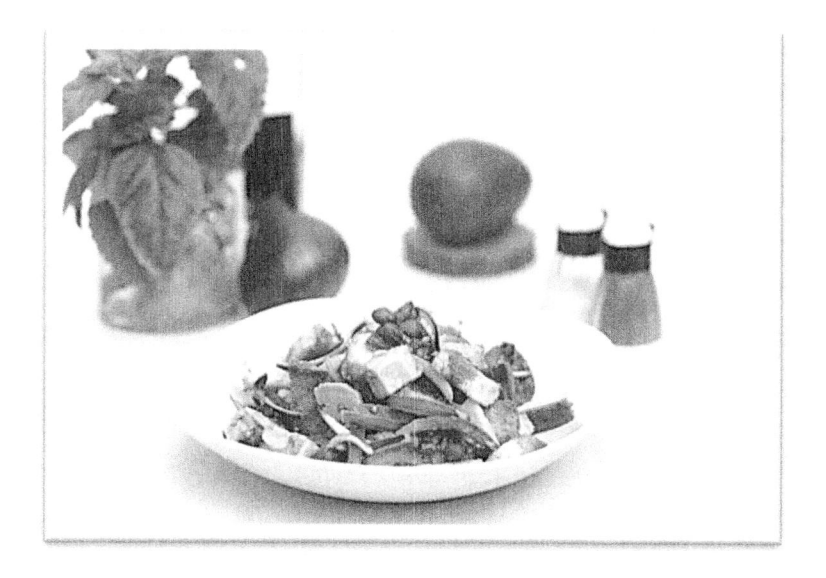

Prep time + Cook time: 10 minutes

Servings: 2

Ingredients

- 2 cups of tomatoes
- 1 crushed garlic clove
- 1 tbsp of drained and rinsed capers

- 1 ripe avocado, peeled and chopped, stoned
- 1 small, very thinly sliced red onion
- 2 slices brown bread
- 2 tbsp of olive oil
- 1 tbsp of red wine vinegar
- A small handful of basil leaves

Instructions

Put the tomatoes in a cup after chopping them. Season with salt and pepper, then toss in the garlic, capers, avocado, and onion. Set aside for 10 mints after thoroughly mixing.

In the meanwhile, break the bread into pieces and put it in a mixing bowl. Pour half of the olive oil than half of the vinegar over the top. Sprinkle tomatoes and basil leaves over the top and drizzle with the remaining oil and vinegar until ready to eat. Before eating, give it a good stir.

4. Quinoa & Stir-Fried Veg

Prep time + Cook time: 30 minutes

Servings: 2

Ingredients

- finely chopped garlic clove

- tbsp of olive oil
- Cut into thin sticks, 2 carrots
- 1 broccoli head
- 1 ⅔ leek, sliced
- ¼ cup of tomatoes
- 1 tsp of tomato purée
- Juice of ½ lemon
- ¼ cup of vegetable stock

Instructions

Cook the quinoa as directed on the package. In the meanwhile, heat 3 tbsp oil in a pan, and add the garlic, then fry for 1 minute. Stir in the carrots, leeks, and broccoli for 2 minutes, or until it is shiny.

Toss in the tomatoes, then mix the stock & tomato purée in a bowl and pour into the pan. Cook for 3 minutes with the lid on. Drain the quinoa and mix it with the remaining oil & lemon juice in a mixing bowl. Spoon the vegetables over top of the vegetables and divide between warm plates.

5. Moroccan Chickpea Soup

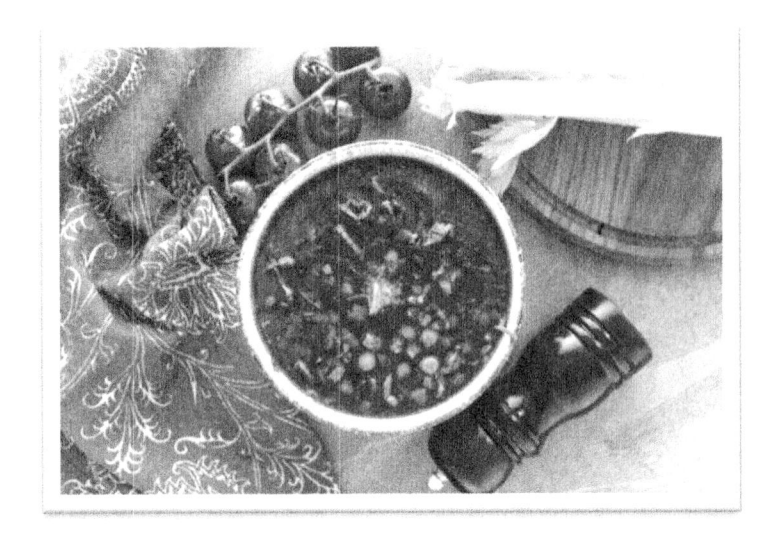

Prep time + Cook time: 25 minutes

Servings: 2

Ingredients

- 1 tbsp of olive oil
- ½ medium chopped onion
- 1 celery chopped sticks
- 1 tsp of ground cumin
- 1 ¼ cups of hot vegetable stock
- 1 cup of chopped tomatoes
- 1 cup of chickpeas, drained and rinsed
- ¼ cup of frozen broad beans

- juice ½ lemon and zest
- bread & coriander to serve

Instructions

In a saucepan, heat the oil and fry the onion & celery for 10 minutes, or until softened. Fry for another minute after adding the cumin.

Add the stock, chickpeas, tomatoes, and black pepper after increasing the heat. Cook for 8 minutes on low heat. Cook for another 2 minutes after adding the broad beans & lemon juice. Serve garnished with lemon zest & coriander.

6. Simple Veggie Wraps

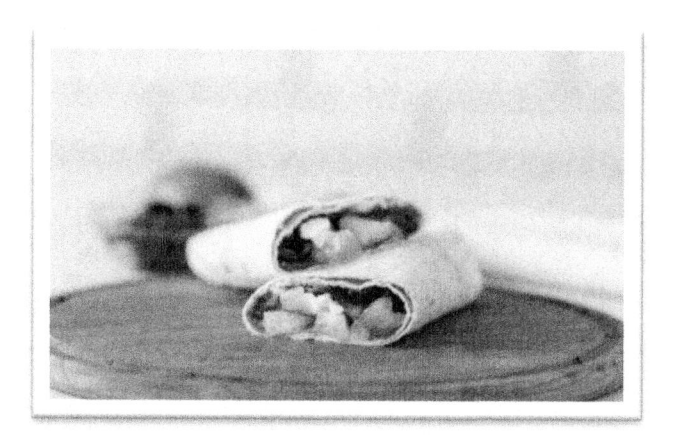

Prep time + Cook time: 10 minutes

Servings: 2

Ingredients

- ½ cup cherry tomatoes
- 6 Kalamata olives
- 1 cucumber
- 2 whole meal large tortilla wraps
- ¼ cup of feta cheese
- 2 tbsp of hummus

Instructions

Remove the stones from the olives, chop the tomatoes, and carve the cucumber into sticks.

Heat the tortillas in a skillet.

Hummus can be spread all over the wrap. Roll up the vegetable mixture in the middle.

7. Carrot, Orange and Avocado Salad

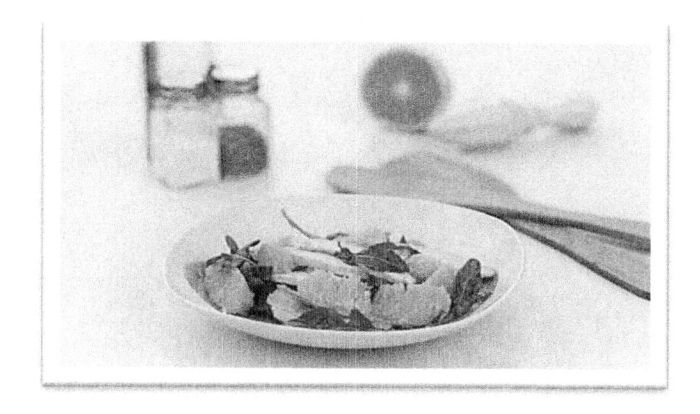

Prep time + Cook time: 5 minutes

Servings: 2

Ingredients

- 2 carrots, sliced and halved lengthways with a peeler
- 1 orange, and juice of 1
- 1 ½ cups of rocket/arugula
- 1 stoned avocado, peeled and sliced
- 1 tbsp of olive oil

Instructions

Cut one of the oranges into segments and combine it with the carrots, rocket/arugula, and avocado in a bowl. Mix the orange juice, zest, and oil in a mixing bowl. Season with salt and pepper and toss through the salad.

8. Mixed Bean Salad

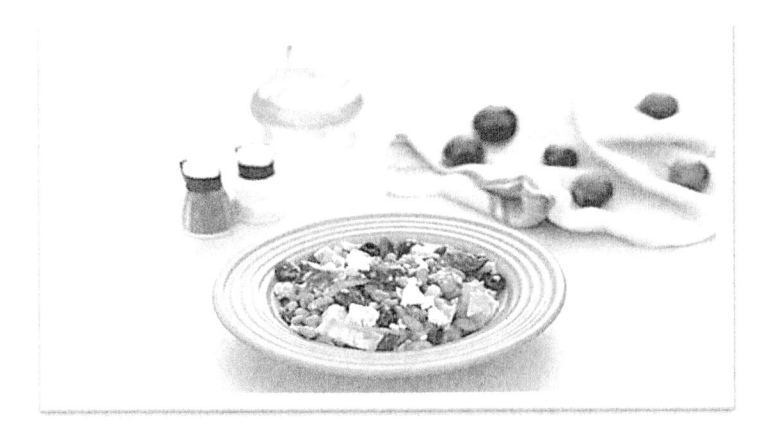

Prep time + cook time: 10 minutes

Servings: 2

Ingredients

- ⅘ cup jar artichoke oil heart
- ½ tbsp of tomato paste sundried
- ½ tsp of red wine vinegar
- 1 cup of drained and rinsed, cannellini beans
- ¾ cup of tomatoes, quartered
- Kalamata black olives, handful
- 2 spring thinly sliced onions(diagonal)
- ⅔ cup of crumbled feta chees

Instructions

Drain the artichoke jar, reserving 1-2 tablespoons of the oil. Stir together the oil, vinegar and sun-dried tomato paste until smooth. Season with salt and pepper to taste.

Chop the artichokes, then place them in a mixing bowl. Mix the cannellini beans, tomatoes, spring olives, onions, and half of the feta cheese in a large mixing bowl. Pour the artichoke oil mixture into a serving bowl and stir to mix. Serve with the leftover feta cheese crumbled on top.

9. Vegetarian Arugula Chickpea Salad

Prep time + Cook time: 25 minutes

Servings: 2

Ingredients

- 15-ounce can of chickpeas beans no-salt-added
- 1 large pitted and diced ripe avocado
- 1/4 cup of red onion diced
- 1 tbsp of lemon juice
- freshly ground black pepper and Salt
- 1 cup of arugula
- 1/4 cup of cucumbers sliced

- 1/4 cup of cooked quinoa
- 1/4 cup of sliced strawberries
- 1/4 cup of cherry tomatoes sliced
- 1 tbsp of crumbled feta
- for drizzling, Balsamic vinegar

Instructions

Drain the chickpeas after rinsing them. Combine the chickpeas & avocado in a medium bowl and mash with

a spoon or potato masher. Mix the onions with lemon juice in a mixing bowl. Salt and pepper to taste. Stir all together thoroughly.

1/2 cup chickpea salad, arugula, cucumbers, quinoa, tomatoes, strawberries, feta, and a drizzle with balsamic vinegar on a plate. Have fun!

The leftover chickpea & avocado salad may be used for anything else.

10. Mixed Berry & Tahini Chia Pudding

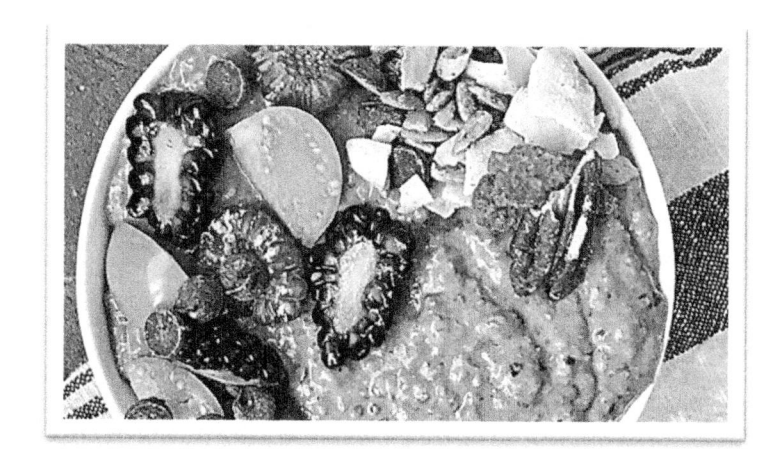

Prep time + Cook time: 15 mints

Servings: 4

Ingredients

- 1 cup of organic coconut milk canned
- 1 cup of frozen mixed berries
- 1/2 cup of milk of preference or unsweetened almond
- 1/4 cup of tahini
- 1/4 cup of **Food Vanilla Collagen**
- 1 tsp of pure vanilla extract
- 1/2 cup of chia seeds
- fruit sweetener, pure stevia, Sugar-free monk or sweetener of choice

Instructions

In a blender container, add frozen berries, coconut milk, milk, and almond or nut-free collagen or Protein, tahini, & vanilla. To taste, adjust the sweetness.

Pulse in the chia seeds before they are just combined.

Cover or securely seal single-serving mason jars with the mixture.

Enable to stay for 10 minutes before shaking or whisking well and cooling overnight or for at least 4 hours.

The Mixed Berry and Tahini Chia Pudding could be kept in the fridge for 3 to 5 days in an airtight container. Warm or cool, with your favorite toppings.

11. Sneaky Liver Burgers

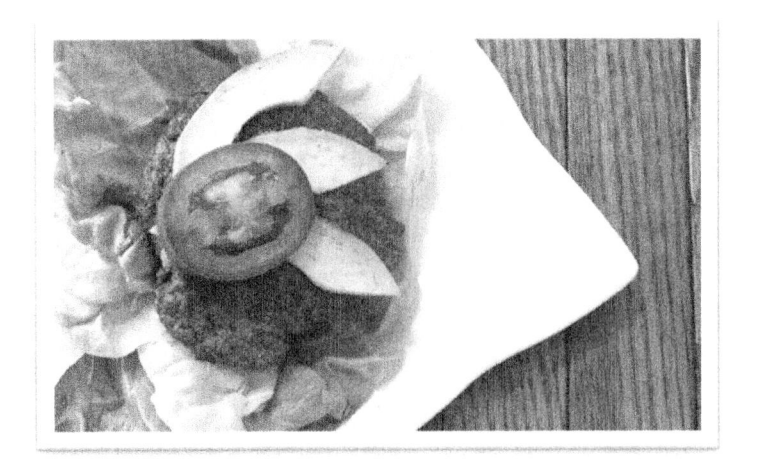

Prep time + Cook time: 15 mints

Servings: 4

Ingredients

- pound of liver
- 1 tbsp of oil (olive oil, coconut oil, or any fat for cooking)
- 1 pound of lean ground beef
- 1 head of iceberg lettuce
- (for seasoning) Sea salt
- (sliced) ripe avocado
- 1 can of hearts of palm
- (for seasoning) Freshly ground black pepper

Instructions

Break the liver into slices and blend until very fine in a food processor.

In a mixing bowl, carefully mix the beef and liver.

After shaping patties with your hands, place them on parchment-lined tray and change the size & thickness to taste. Using salt and pepper, season to taste.

Refrigerate for 10 minutes to firm up the patties.

Over medium-high heat, melt the butter in a large

saucepan. If the oil has reached the desired temperature, add the patties. Be sure the pan isn't crowded.

Brown all sides of the patties in an oven.

Tear off big bits of lettuce to make "buns."

Place the patty, palm hearts, and avocado around lettuce leaves to make the "burger."

Serve with your favorite extra toppings. These burgers go well with a side of garlic-roasted sweet potato fries.

12. Grass-Fed Beef Liver Pate

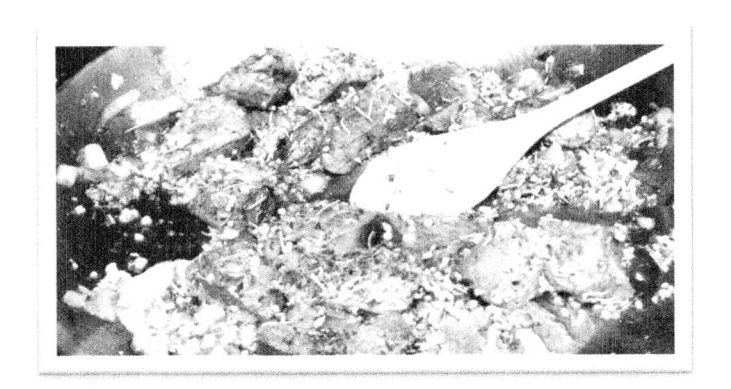

Prep time + Cook time: 15

Servings: 10

Ingredients

- 1 medium-size onion
- 1 pound of beef liver grass-fed (thin slices)

- 1 cup of coconut oil (can use olive oil, lard or duck Fat, bacon fat)
- 1 tbsp of apple cider vinegar (red wine vinegar or balsamic, also taste great)
- 2-3 tbsps of minced garlic
- 1 1/2 tbsps of fresh rosemary
- salt & pepper for taste
- 1 tbsp of fresh thyme

Instructions

2 tablespoons coconut oil (or desired fat) for frying liver and onions until onions are caramelized and the liver is cooked through.

Mix the garlic, cider vinegar, thyme, rosemary, and Superfood Turmeric in a mixing bowl.

Cook for another few minutes before the vinegar's liquid has been reduced.

Remove from heat and set aside for 5 minutes to cool.

1/4 to 1/2 cup of oil can be added to a food processor.

Mix thoroughly, adding the remaining oil if appropriate until the mixture is moist and fluffy.

Portion into storage containers.

6.4 Fatty Liver Friendly Dinner Recipes

1. Moussaka

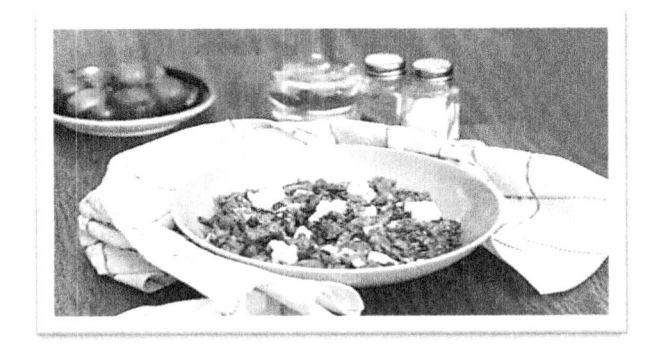

Prep time + Cook time: 30 minutes

Servings: 2

Ingredients

- ½ finely chopped onion
- 1 tbsp of extra virgin olive oil
- 1 finely chopped garlic clove
- 1 cup of chopped tomatoes
- 9 oz. of mince lean beef
- 1 tbsp of tomato purée
- 1 cup of chickpeas
- 1 tsp of ground cinnamon
- ⅔ cup of crumbled feta cheese

- Brown bread, for serving
- Mint (fresh)

Instructions

In a pan, heat the oil. Fry the onion and garlic until they are fluffy. Cook for 3-4 minutes, or until the mince is browned.

Season with salt and pepper after adding the tomatoes, tomato purée, and cinnamon to the pan. Allow 20 minutes for the mince to simmer. Halfway through, add the chickpeas.

Over the mince, sprinkle the feta and mint. Serve with toasted bread as a side dish.

2. Tomato Baked Eggs

Prep time + Cook time: 25 minutes

Servings: 2

Ingredients

- 2 chopped red onions
- 1 tbsp of olive oil
- 1 deseeded & chopped red chili
- A small bunch coriander, leaves and stalks separately chopped

- 1 sliced garlic clove
- 4 cups of cherry tomatoes
- 1 brown bread, for serving
- 4 large eggs

Instructions

In a frying pan with lid, heat the oil and cook the onions, chili, garlic and coriander stalks until tender, around 5 minutes. Simmer for 8 to10 minutes after adding the tomatoes.

Make 4 dips in sauce with the back of a spoon, then crack an egg in each one. Cover the pan and cook for 6-8 minutes over low heat or until the eggs are cooked to your taste. Serve with bread, and coriander leaves sprinkled on top.

3. Salmon with Potatoes & Corn Salad

Prep time + Cook time: 30 minutes

Servings: 2

Ingredients

- sweetcorn cob
- ⅓ cups of baby new potatoes
- salmon fillets skinless

- 1 tbsp of vinegar red wine
- ⅓ cup of tomatoes
- 1 tbsp of olive oil extra-virgin
- 1 tbsp of finely chopped capers
- Bunch of finely chopped scallions or spring onions,
- basil leaves, a handful

Instructions

Cook potatoes until soft in boiling water, then add corn for the last 5 minutes. Drain and set aside to cool.

To make the dressing, mix the oil, shallot, capers, basil, vinegar, and seasoning in a mixing bowl.

Preheat the grill to high heat. Cook for 7-8 minutes, skinned side down, with some dressing on salmon. Place tomatoes on a plate, sliced. Cut the corn from cob and place it on the plate with the potatoes. Drizzle the leftover dressing over the salmon.

4. Spiced Carrot & Lentil Soup

Prep time + Cook time: 25 minutes

Servings: 2

Ingredients

- pinch chili flakes
- 1 tsp of cumin seeds
- 1 tbsp of olive oil
- ⅓ cup of split red lentils
- cups washed & coarsely grated carrots
- ¼ cups of hot vegetable stock
- to serve Greek yogurt
- ¼ cup of milk

Instructions

Dry fry that cumin seeds & chili flakes in a large saucepan for 1 minute. Set aside about half of the seeds after scooping them out with a spoon. Bring the oil, carrots, lentils, stock, and milk to a boil in the pan. Cook for 15 minutes, or until the lentils are softened and swollen.

Using a stick blender or a food processor, puree the soup until creamy. Season to taste, then top with a dollop of yogurt (Greek) and a sprinkling of toasted spices set aside.

5. Med Chicken, Quinoa & Greek Salad

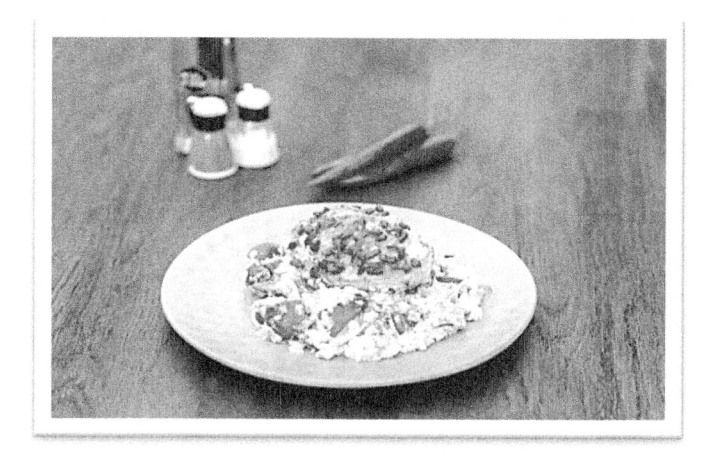

Prep time + Cook time: 20 minutes

Servings: 2

Ingredients

- ½ deseeded & finely chopped red chili
- ⅗ cup of quinoa
- 1 crushed garlic clove
- 1 tbsp of extra-virgin olive oil
- 2 breasts of chicken
- ¾ cup of roughly chopped tomatoes
- ½ finely sliced red onion
- pitted black kalamata olives, a handful
- ½ cup of crumbled feta cheese

- zest ½ lemon and juice
- mint leaves, small bunch, chopped

Instructions

Cook the quinoa according to the package directions, then clean and drain thoroughly.

In the meantime, toss the chicken fillets with some seasoning, garlic and chili in olive oil. Cook for 3 to 4 minutes on either side in a hot skillet or until cooked through. Place the chicken on a plate and put it aside.

In a mixing bowl, mix the tomatoes, olives, feta, onion and mint. Toss in the quinoa that has been baked. Season to taste with the remaining olive oil, zest and lemon juice. Put the chicken on top and serve.

6. Mediterranean Beet Salad

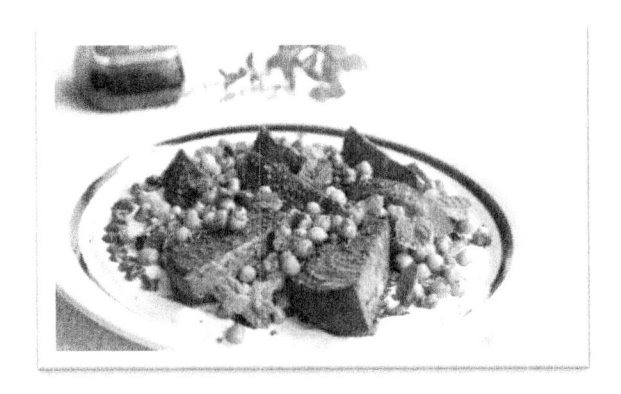

Prep time + Cook time: 40 minutes

Servings: 2

Ingredients

- 4 medium or 8 raw baby beetroots, scrubbed
- ½ tbsp of sumac
- ½ tbsp of ground cumin
- 2 cups of drained and rinsed chickpeas
- 2 tbsp of olive oil
- ½ tsp of lemon zest
- ½ tsp of lemon juice
- ½ cup of Greek yogurt
- 1 tbsp of harissa paste
- 1 tsp of rushed red chili flakes
- Chopped mint leaves to serve

Instructions

Preheat the oven to 220°F/200°F fan/gas 7. Beetroots may be halved or quartered based on their scale. Mix the spices in a bowl. Mix the chickpeas and beets with the oil in a large baking tray. Season with salt and toss in the spices. Re-mix the ingredients. 30 minutes of roasting

Mix the lemon juice and zest with the yogurt when the

vegetables are frying. Swirl in the harissa and transfer to a bowl. Add the beetroot on top.

7. Edgy Veggie Wraps

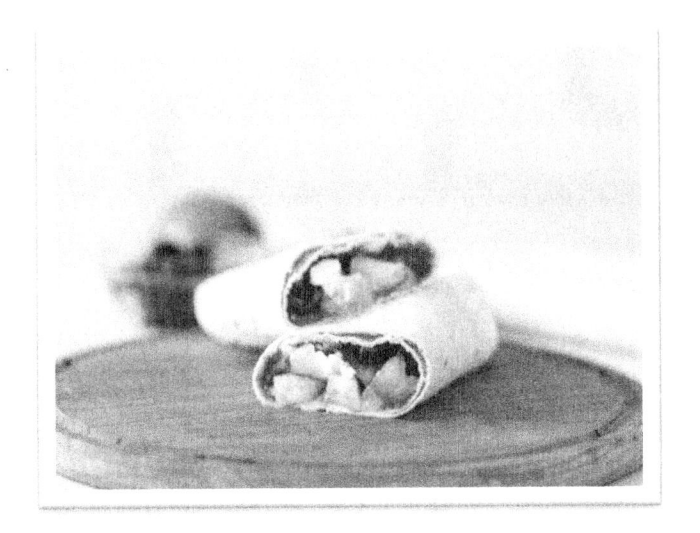

Prep time + Cook time: 10 minutes

Servings: 2

Ingredients

- ½ cup cherry tomatoes
- 6 Kalamata olives
- 1 cucumber
- 2 whole meal large tortilla wraps
- ¼ cup of feta cheese
- 2 tbsp of hummus

Instructions

Remove the stones from the olives, chop the tomatoes, and carve the cucumber into sticks.

Heat the tortillas in a skillet.

Hummus can be spread all over the wrap. Roll up the vegetable mixture in the middle.

8. Spicy Tomato Baked Eggs

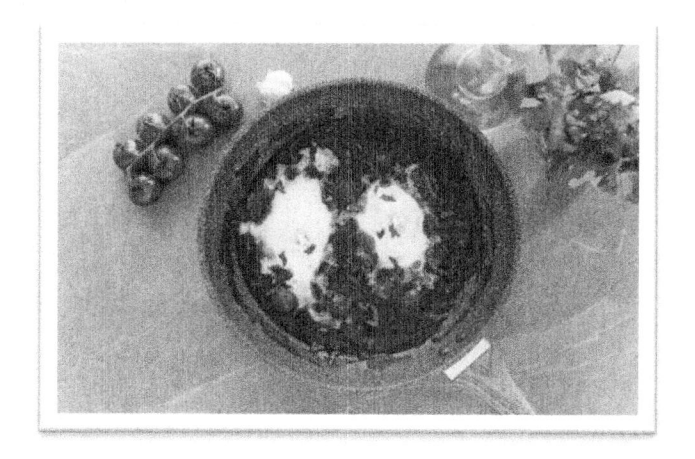

Prep time + Cook time: 25 minutes

Servings: 2

Ingredients

- 1 tbsp of olive oil
- 2 chopped red onions
- 1 deseeded & chopped red chili

- 1 sliced garlic clove
- Small bunch coriander, leaves and stalks separately chopped
- 4 cups of cherry tomatoes
- 4 large eggs
- to serve, brown bread

Instructions

In a frying pan with lid, heat the oil and cook the onions, garlic, chili and coriander stalks until tender, around 5 minutes. Simmer for 8-10 mints after adding the tomatoes.

Create 4 dips in the sauce with the back of a spoon, then crack an egg in each one. Cover the pan and cook for 6-8 minutes over low heat or until the eggs are cooked to your taste. Serve with bread, and coriander leaves sprinkled on top.

9. Salmon with Potatoes & Corn Salad

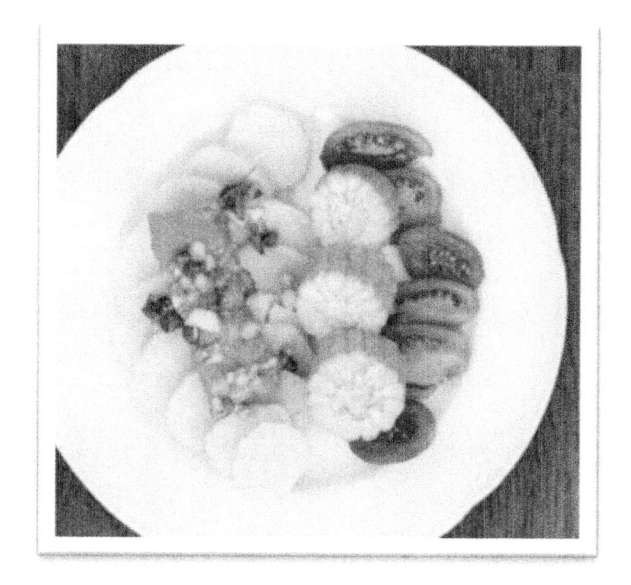

Prep time + Cook time: 30 minutes

Servings: 2

Ingredients

- sweetcorn cob
- ⅓ cups of baby new potatoes
- salmon fillets skinless
- 1 tbsp of vinegar red wine
- ⅓ cup of tomatoes
- 1 tbsp of olive oil extra-virgin
- 1 tbsp of finely chopped capers

- Bunch of finely chopped scallions or spring onions,
- basil leaves, a handful

Instructions

Cook potatoes until soft in boiling water, then add corn for the last 5 minutes. Drain and set aside to cool.

To make the dressing, mix the oil, shallot, capers, basil, vinegar, and seasoning in a mixing bowl.

Preheat the grill to high heat. Cook for 7-8 minutes, skinned side down, with some dressing on salmon. Place tomatoes on a plate, sliced. Cut the corn from the cob and place it on the plate with the potatoes. Drizzle the leftover dressing over the salmon.

10. Spiced Carrot & Lentil Soup

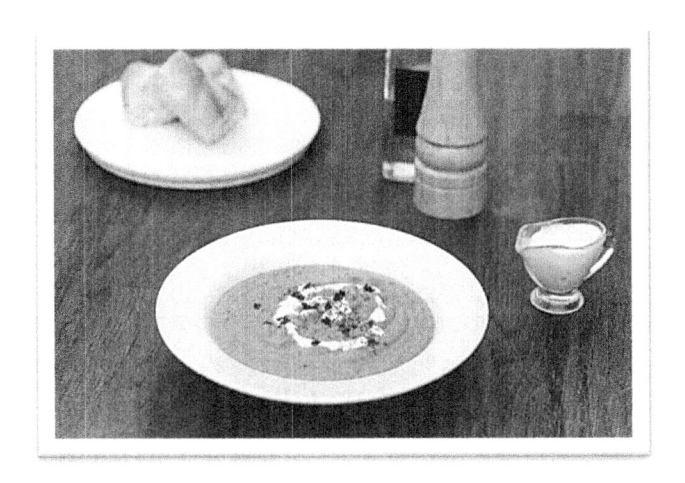

Prep time + Cook time: 25 minutes

Servings: 2

Ingredients

- pinch chili flakes
- 1 tsp of cumin seeds
- 1 tbsp of olive oil
- ⅓ cup of split red lentils
- cups washed & coarsely grated carrots
- ¼ cups of hot vegetable stock
- to serve Greek yogurt
- ¼ cup of milk

Instructions

Dry fry that cumin seeds & chili flakes in a large saucepan for 1 minute. Set aside about half of the seeds after scooping them out with a spoon. Bring the oil, carrots, lentils, stock, and milk to a boil in the pan. Cook for 15 minutes, or until the lentils are softened and swollen.

Using a stick blender or a food processor, puree the soup until creamy. Season to taste, then top with a dollop of Greek yogurt and a sprinkling of toasted spices that were set aside.

11. Mediterranean-style grilled salmon

Prep time + Cook time: 20 mints

Servings: 1

Ingredients

- tbsp of chopped fresh parsley
- 4 tbsps of chopped fresh basil
- tbsp of minced garlic
- 4 salmon fillets, 5 ounces each
- tbsps of lemon juice
- Black pepper, to taste
- thin lemon slices
- chopped green olives

Instructions

In a barbecue grill, create a fire, or heat a broiler or gas grill. Spray the grill rack gently with cooking spray away from the heat source. 4 to 6 inches away from the heat source, position the cooking rack.

Combine the basil, parsley, chopped garlic, and lemon juice in a small bowl. Cooking spray can be sprayed on the fish. Season with black pepper to taste. Similar quantities of the herb-garlic mixture should be added to each fillet. Place the fish on the grill with the herb side down. Preheat the grill to high. Turn the fish over and put on aluminum foil when the edges turn white around 3 or 4 minutes. Reduce the heat or transfer the fish to the cooler section of the grill. Grill before an instant-read thermometer into the thickest part of fish reads 145 F, and the fish is opaque when examined with the tip of a knife (about 4 minutes longer).

Place the salmon on warmed plates after removing it from the bowl. Serve with green olives & lemon slices as garnish.

12. Spinach & Mushroom Quesadilla

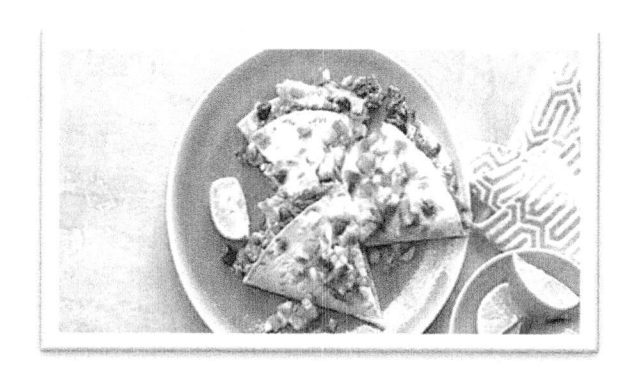

Prep time + Cook time: 25 mints

Servings: 2

Ingredients

- ½ cup of sliced mushrooms (40 g)

- 1 tbsp of olive oil
- 2 cloves of garlic
- Salt and pepper to taste
- 3 cups of fresh spinach (120 g)
- 3 eggs
- 1 cup of mozzarella cheese shredded, double if 2 quesadillas
- 2 large flour tortillas
- ½ cup of parmesan cheese shredded (60 g), double if 2 quesadillas

Instructions

Allow the oil to heat up in a skillet before adding the garlic and mushrooms. Cook, sometimes stirring until the mushrooms fully softened and caramelized somewhat.

Cook, constantly stirring, until the spinach has wilted.

Scramble the eggs and veggies together. Season with salt & pepper and continue to stir until it is thoroughly cooked. Remove the pan from the heat and put it aside.

Place the tortilla in a skillet and cover half of it with a layer of both kinds of cheese.

Add the scramble to the tortilla, cover with more cheese,

and fold it in two.

Over medium heat, cook for 6 minutes, flipping halfway through.

Serve with salsa & fresh parsley on top.

Have fun!

13. One-Skillet Chicken with Green Olives and Tomatoes

Prep time + Cook Time: 30 mints,

Servings: 3-4

Ingredients:

- 4 Equal size skinless, boneless chicken breasts
- 2 tbsp. of garlic paste or minced garlic
- Salt & pepper
- 1 tbsp. of divided dried oregano,
- Olive oil extra virgin private reserve
- ½ cup of wine dry white
- Juice of 1 large lemon,
- ½ cup of chicken broth
- 1 cup of red onion finely chopped
- 1 ½ cup of tomatoes well diced

- ¼ cup of green olives sliced
- A handful of chopped & stems removed, fresh parsley,
- Feta cheese crumbled

Instructions:

Pat and rinse the chicken breasts. Create three slits along each side of that chicken breast.

On both sides, spread the garlic; add some garlic into the slits you have created. On both ends, season chicken breasts with salt, pepper & 1/2 of the dried oregano.

Heat 2 tsps. of olive oil in a large cast-iron skillet over medium-high heat. In all ends, brown the chicken. , Add the white wine, lemon juice & chicken broth and let it decrease by 1/2. Sprinkle on top of the remaining oregano. Decrease to medium heat. Cover with a lid, or foil securely. Cook for 10-15 mints and switch the chicken over once (the chicken's inner temperature should exceed 165 degrees F.)

Uncover & top with the chopped onions, tomatoes & olives that have been diced. Cover it for just 3 mints again. Finally, add the feta and parsley cheese. Serve with light pasta, couscous, or rice.

14. Mediterranean-Style Fish Soup Recipe

Prep time + Cook Time: 25 mints,

Servings: 2

Ingredients:

- 1 ½ tsp. of coriander
- 1 tsp. of cumin
- 1 tsp. of Aleppo pepper flakes
- ½ tsp. of paprika
- ¾ tsp. of turmeric
- 1 ½ lbs. fish fillet moderately firm, use a combination of red snapper & sea bass, cut in chunks
- Kosher salt & black pepper
- olive oil Extra virgin
- 1 chopped red onion,
- 2, chopped
- 1 chopped red bell pepper,
- 4 minced garlic cloves
- 1 28- oz. can of whole tomatoes
- ½ cup of white wine

- 4 cups of chicken stock or vegetable stock, low-sodium preferably
- 1 cup of packed fresh chopped cilantro
- 1 cup of packed fresh chopped parsley
- 3 chopped green onions (white & green parts both)
- juice of 1 lemon

Instructions:

Mix up the spices in a small bowl.

A reasonable pinch of kosher salt & black pepper and 2 or 3 tsps. of the spice mixture is added to the fish seasoning, toss to coat.

Heat 3 tbsp extra virgin olive oil in a big pot or Dutch oven over medium-high heat. Add the onions, garlic, bell peppers, and celery. Cook for 5 mints just till the time vegetables soften, tossing continuously. Using a healthy pinch of kosher salt & black pepper to season. Apply the rest of the blend of spices.

Add the tomatoes, the white wine & the broth of the chicken. Get it to a boil, then lower the temperature to medium-low heat. Cover that pot part-way and give 20 mints to simmer.

Add the fish, then cook for 4 - 5 mints or until the fish is completely cooked (don't over-cook that fish, and remember to continue to cook in the hot broth even to remove from the heat).

Stir in the cilantro, parsley & green onions. Finish with the juice of the lemon. And Serve Immediately

15. Avocado with Cucumber Quinoa Salad

Prep time + Cook time: 10 mints

Servings: 4

Ingredients

- 1 cucumber large size
- 1 avocado large size
- 1 cup of cooked quinoa
- 1/2 cup of red onion diced
- 1/2 - 3/4 dressing batch
- For garnish Hemp seeds (optional)

For Dressing:

- 1/3 cup of water
- 1/4 cup of raw cashews
- 1/4 cup of parsley
- 1/4 cup of cilantro

- 1/4 cup of spinach
- 2 scallions
- 1 lime for Juice
- 2 tsps of soy sauce
- Salt & pepper

Instructions

Remove the pit from the avocado and cut it in half. Scoop into a big mixing bowl and cut into bite-sized portions. Cucumbers can be sliced lengthwise down the center. Then split it into three long, equal strips. The cucumber can then be chopped into cubes and added to the mixing cup.

Place aside the quinoa and onion.

In a high-powered blender, combine the water, cashews, herbs, spinach, lime juice, scallions and soy sauce. Blend on high speed until the mixture is thick and fluffy. Season with salt & pepper to taste, if necessary.

Toss around half to three-quarters of the dressing into the mixing bowl to blend. If you like to incorporate more dressing, go ahead and do so!

Serve with hemp seeds sprinkled on top.

16. Farfalle with Tuna, Lemon, and Fennel

Prep time + Cook Time: 20 mints

Servings: 2

Ingredients:

- 6 oz. farfalle (bow-tie) pasta of dried whole grain
- 1 (5 ounces) can of tuna solid white (oil-packed)
- Olive oil
- 1 cup of thinly sliced fennel (1 medium bulb)
- 2 minced garlic, cloves
- ½ tsp. of red pepper crushed
- ¼ tsp. of salt
- 2 (14.5 oz.) cans of undrained diced tomatoes no-salt-added,
- 1 tsp. of finely shredded lemon peel,
- 2 tbsps. of fresh Italian parsley snipped (flat-leaf)

Instructions:

Cook pasta, omitting salt according to box **Instructions**; rinse. Put the pasta back into the pan; cover & keep warm. In the meanwhile, rinse the tuna & reserving oil. To weigh 3 tbsps. Overall, add enough olive oil if necessary. Tuna flakes; set back.

Heat the 3 tbsps. of the reserved oil in a medium saucepan over medium heat. Add fennel; cook, stirring regularly, for 3 mints. Add the garlic, salt & crushed red pepper; cook and mix until the garlic is golden, or around 1 minute.

Stir the tomatoes in. Get it to a boil; lower the flame. Simmer for 5 to 6 mints, uncovered, or before the mixture begins to thicken. Stir in the tuna; simmer, uncovered, around 1 minute more or until the tuna is thoroughly cooked.

Pour the mixture of tuna over the pasta; stir to blend gently. Sprinkle with parsley & lemon peel for each serving.

17. Mediterranean Portobello Mushroom Pizzas with Arugula Salad

Prep time + Cook Time: 45 mints

Servings: 4

Ingredients:

- 8 cups of large gills removed Portobello mushroom
- 2 tbsps. of olive oil + 1 tsp., divided
- ½ tsp. of ground pepper
- ½ cup of tomato sauce or pizza sauce
- 2 cups of chopped baby spinach lightly packed,
- ½ cup of chopped sun-dried tomatoes (about 8 tomatoes),
- 1 (14 oz.) can of artichoke hearts, rinsed & chopped
- ½ cup of part-skim mozzarella cheese shredded
- ¼ cup of feta cheese crumbled
- ½ tsp. of Italian seasoning dried
- 1 tbsp. of lemon juice
- 2 cups of baby arugula lightly packed
- ¼ cup of thinly sliced fresh basil leaves,

Instructions:

Preheat the oven to 400°F. Line a large foil baking sheet and put a wire rack upon that. With 1 tbsp, brush tops to Portobello caps Oil, then position them on the rack, underside-up. For 10 mints, roast. For 5 more mints, flip and roast.

Take the Portobello's out of the oven and turn them back over gently so that undersides become up. Season with tsp. 1/4. With pepper. Spread out 1 tbsp. So each cap has sauce inside. Divide the caps with spinach, sun-dried tomatoes, mozzarella, artichokes & feta. Sprinkle with Italian seasoning. Put the Portobello's back in the oven and bake for 10 - 15 mints till the time cheese is melted and begins to brown.

In the meantime, mix the remaining 1 tbsp. And plus 1 tsp. Oil, 1/8 tsp. remaining. Pepper, & lemon juice in medium bowl, Add the arugula and coat with a toss.

Garnish with basil on the Portobello pizzas and use the arugula salad to serve with.

18. Cauliflower, Pancetta & Olive Spaghetti

Prep time + Cook Time: 30 mints

Servings: 4

Ingredients:

- 8 oz. spaghetti whole-wheat
- 1 tbsp. of olive oil extra-virgin
- 4 cups of cauliflower finely chopped
- ¼ cup of pancetta diced
- 2 cloves of finely chopped garlic,
- ½ cup of white dry wine
- 8 sliced pitted Kalamata olives,
- ¼ cup of roasted red peppers finely chopped
- 1 tbsp. of butter
- ¼ cup of flat-leaf parsley chopped
- ¼ tsp. of salt
- ¼ tsp. of ground pepper

Instructions:

For 1 minute less than the package **Instructions**, cook pasta. Place aside 1 cup of pasta water, and then drain.

Meanwhile, over medium heat, heat the oil in a large skillet. Cook the cauliflower & pancetta and occasionally stirring for about 10 mints until the cauliflower starts to brown. Add garlic and cook for 30 seconds, continue stirring. Stir in the wine, heat up to high, and cook until almost evaporated, stirring occasionally around 2 mints. Stir in the peppers, butter, and olives. Add the pasta together with the reserved cooking water; simmer for 1 to 2 more mints until the water is about to evaporate. Stir in the parsley, pepper & salt.

19. Seared Cod with Spinach-Lemon Sauce

Prep time + Cook Time: 25 mints

Servings: 4

Ingredients:

- 1 5-oz of package baby spinach
- ½ cup of fresh parsley sprigs lightly packed
- 3 tbsps. of water
- 4 tsps. of orange juice
- 4 tsps. of lemon juice
- ½ tsp. of salt, divided
- 1 quartered garlic clove,

- ½ tsp. of ground pepper, divided
- 1 ¼ lb. of cod, cut in 4 portions
- ¼ tsp. of red pepper crushed
- ¼ cup of sliced toasted almonds
- 1 tbsp. of canola oil or grape-seed oil

Instructions:

Place the spinach and water in a bowl that is suitable for microwaves. Cover and poke a few gaps in it with plastic wrap. Microwave on high, about 2 mints, before wilted.

In a mixer, combine the wilted spinach (and any leftover water), lemon juice, parsley, garlic, orange juice, 1/4 tsp. of each salt & pepper and crushed red pepper till creamy. Just put it back.

Sprinkle the remaining 1/4 of a tsp. of salt & pepper with the cod.

Heat oil over medium-high heat in large nonstick skillet. Cook the cod, rotating once, till it is golden brown and cooked through, for a total of 5 to 7 mints. Transfer in a plate; keep the tent warm with foil.

Pour that reserved sauce in to pan and cook until slightly thickened, stirring occasionally, for around 1 minute. Serve the fish sprinkled with almonds on top of the sauce.

20. Shrimp Piccata with Zucchini Noodles

Prep time + Cook Time: 35 mints

Servings: 4

Ingredients:

- 5-6 medium-size trimmed zucchini (about 2 1/2 pounds),
- ½ tsp. of salt
- 2 tbsps. of olive oil extra-virgin, divided
- 2 tbsps. of butter
- 2 minced cloves of garlic
- 1 lbs. of raw shrimp peeled and deveined, tails left if desired (21-25 count)
- 1 tbsp. of cornstarch
- 1 cup of chicken broth low-sodium
- ¼ cup of lemon juice
- ⅓ cup of white wine
- 3 tbsps. of rinsed capers
- 2 tbsps. of fresh parsley chopped

Instructions:

Cut the zucchini lengthwise into long, thin strands or strips using a spiral vegetable slicer or a vegetable peeler. Stop in the middle when you reach the seeds (seeds make the noodles apart). In a colander, place the zucchini noodles and toss them with salt. Drain for 15 - 30 mints, then squeeze gently to remove any excess water.

In the meantime, over medium-high heat, heat the butter and 1 tbsp. of oil in a large skillet. Add the garlic and cook for 30 seconds, stirring. Add the shrimp and cook for 1 minute, stirring.

In a small bowl, whisk the broth and cornstarch together. You can add wine, lemon juice & capers to the shrimp. Simmer, stirring occasionally, 4 - 5 mints, till the time shrimp has just cooked through. Simply remove from the heat.

In a large nonstick skillet, heat the remaining 1 tbsp. of oil over med- high heat. Add the zucchini noodles and toss gently for about 3 mints, till hot. Serve the shrimp & sauce, sprinkled with parsley, over the zucchini noodles.

21. Greek Stuffed Portobello Mushrooms

Prep time + Cook Time: 25 mints

Servings: 4

Ingredients:

- 3 tbsps. of olive oil extra-virgin, divided

- 1 minced of clove garlic,
- ¼ tsp. of salt
- ½ tsp. of ground pepper, divided
- 4 (about 14 ounces) Portobello mushrooms, stems & gills removed, wiped clean
- 1 cup of spinach chopped
- ⅓ cup of crumbled feta cheese
- ½ cup of quartered cherry tomatoes
- 1 tbsp. of fresh oregano chopped
- 2 tbsps. of Kalamata olives sliced & pitted

Instructions:

Preheat the oven to 400°F.

In a small bowl, combine 2 tbsps. of oil, 1/4 of a tsp. of pepper & salt, garlic, Coat the mushrooms all over with an oil mixture using a silicone brush. Place on the large

rimmed baking sheet, then bake for 8 -10 mints till the time mushrooms are mostly soft.

In the meantime, in a medium bowl, combine the spinach, feta, tomato, olives, oregano, and remaining 1 tbsp. of oil. Remove from the oven once the mushrooms have softened and filled with spinach mixture. Bake for about 10 mints till the tomatoes have wilted.

22. Swordfish with Olives, Capers & Tomatoes over Polenta

Prep time + Cook Time: 45 mints

Servings: 4

Ingredients:

- ½ tsp. of salt, divided
- 2 ½ cups of water
- ½ cup of regular yellow polenta or cornmeal
- 4 medium diced stalks, celery,
- 1 tbsp. of olive oil extra-virgin
- 2 minced cloves of garlic
- ¼ cup of green olives, such as Cerignola or Sicilian colossal, pitted & coarsely chopped, rinsed,
- 1 (15 oz.) can of diced tomatoes no-salt-added
- 3 tbsps. of fresh basil chopped
- 1 tbsp. of rinsed capers,
- Pinch of red pepper crushed
- ⅛ tsp. of ground pepper
- 1 lb. of swordfish, cut in 4 steaks
- for garnish, use Fresh basil

Instructions:

In a medium-size saucepan over a high flame, put 2 cups of water to a boil. Add 1/4 tsp. of salt. Slowly pour in a gentle stream of cornmeal (or polenta), stirring quickly with a wooden spoon to prevent lumps. Cook for about 3 mints, stirring, before the mixture begins to thicken.

Lower the flame to a moderate simmer. Cook, and stirring every 5 mints, 20 to 25 mints, until the polenta is easily separated from the sides of the pan. Crush some lumps into the side of the pan when cooking. To stir, include 1/2 cup of water if the polenta gets too thick. A thick porridge should be close to the final texture. Remove from the heat and, to keep warm, cover.

In the meantime, over medium heat, heat the oil in a large skillet. Add celery; cook, stirring often, for about 5 mints, till tender. Add garlic; cook for 30 seconds till it is aromatic, not browned. Also include the tomatoes, basil, capers, olives, ground pepper, crushed red pepper, and remaining 1/4 tsp salt. Cover, lower the heat to a minimum, and cook for 5 mints to boil.

In the simmering sauce, place the swordfish steaks. Cover and cook for 10 to 15 mints, till the time fish is thoroughly cooked.

Spoon the polenta to a large serving platter to serve. Arrange that fish over the polenta, cover it with the sauce, and, if needed, garnish it with fresh basil.

23. Greek Burgers with Herb-Feta Sauce

Prep time + Cook Time: 25 mints

Servings: 4

Ingredients:

- 1 cup of plain Greek yogurt nonfat
- ¼ cup of feta cheese crumbled
- ¼ tsp. of lemon zest
- 3 tbsps. of fresh oregano chopped, divided
- ¾ tsp. of salt, divided
- 2 tsps. of lemon juice
- 1 lb. ground beef or ground lamb
- 1 small red onion
- ½ tsp. of ground pepper
- 2, split and warmed, halved whole-wheat pitas,
- 1 plum sliced tomato,
- 1 cup sliced of cucumber

Instructions:

Preheat the medium-high grill or preheat the broiler to high.

In a small bowl, mix the feta, yogurt, 1 tbsp. oregano, lemon juice, lemon zest, and 1/4 of a tsp. of salt.

To get 1/4 cup, cut out 1/4-inch-thick pieces of onion. To get 1/4 cup, finely chop some more onion. (For further use, reserve any leftover onion.) In a large bowl, mix the minced onion and meat with the remaining 2 tsps. of oregano and 1/2 tsp salt and pepper each. Four oval patties, around 4 inches by 3 inches,

Broil or Grill the burgers, turning once, till 160 degrees F is registered by an instant-read thermometer, 4–6 mints per side. And Serve with the sauce, cucumber, onion slices, and tomato in pita halves.

24. Bean Mash with Grilled Vegetables

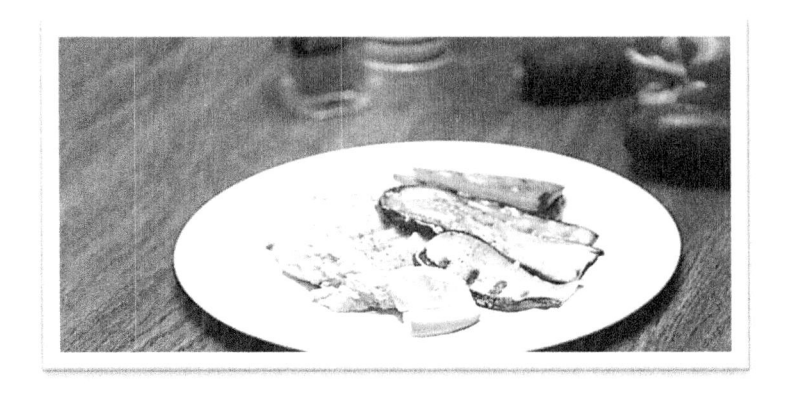

Prep time + Cook time: 40 minutes

Servings: 2

Ingredients

- 1 deseeded & quartered pepper
- 1 sliced lengthways aubergine
- 2 sliced lengthways courgettes
- 2 tbsp of olive oil

   For mash

- 2 cups of rinsed haricot beans
- 1 crushed garlic clove
- 1 tbsp of chopped coriander
- ½ cup of vegetable stock

Instructions

Preheat the grill to high. Brush the vegetables gently with oil and arrange them on a grill pan. Grill until finely browned on one hand, then flip and grill until tender on the other.

Meanwhile, mix the beans, garlic, and stock in a pan. Carry to a simmer, then reduce to a low heat and cook for 10 minutes, uncovered. Using a potato masher, mash the potatoes. Divide and mash the vegetables between two bowls, then drizzle with oil and season with black pepper & coriander.

25. Herbed Chicken and Vegetable Skillet

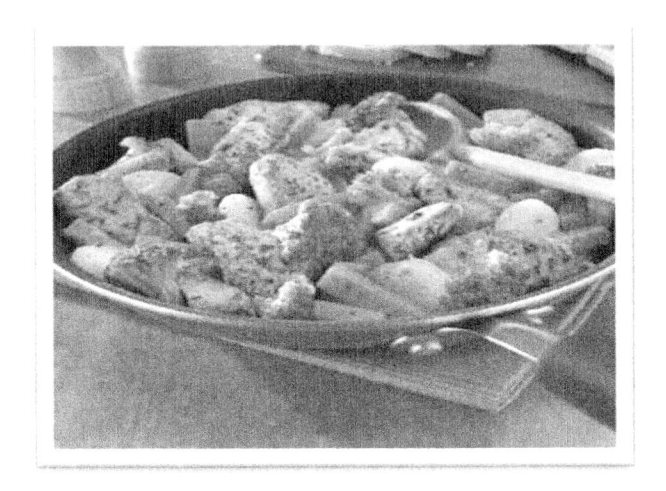

Prep time + Cook time: 35 mints

Servings: 5

Ingredients

- 3 tbsps of butter
- 4 boneless skinless (5-ounce) chicken breasts, cut into half-inch wide strips
- tsp of salt
- tsp of thyme leaves dried
- ¼ tsp of pepper
- ¼ cup of water

- 1 bag (16-ounce) frozen vegetable combination (carrots, broccoli, and water chestnuts)

Instructions

In a 10-inch skillet, melt the butter until it bubbles, then add the chicken strips, pepper, thyme leaves, and salt. Cook, stirring regularly, for 5-6 minutes over medium-high heat, or until chicken seems to be no longer pink. Mix the water and vegetable mixture in a large mixing bowl. Cook, stirring regularly, for another 4-5 minutes, or until the mixture comes to a simmer.

Reduce to a medium heat setting. Cook, covered, for 10-12 minutes or till vegetables are crisp-tender, stirring periodically.

Conclusion

Researchers have looked into the connection between nutrients/food/meals, eating habits, and NAFLD in the last decade. Nutritional study into the treatment of NAFLD patients is a big problem. This is especially significant because behavioral changes such as diet, exercise, and weight reduction are successful in NAFLD treatment. Long-term consequences of calorie-restricted diets result in improvements in many NAFLD characteristics. While further research is required to explain this topic, the diet's basic macronutrient content appears to be less significant. Hypocaloric foods, including high fat and low carbohydrate but low fat and high carbohydrate, have been shown to minimize liver lipids equally. The Western diet is linked to a higher incidence of NAFLD, while the Mediterranean diet improves steatosis even in weight loss. One of the most challenging aspects of researching diet and NAFLD is the disease's gradual development. To track histopathological endpoints, prospective long-term trials of liver biopsies are also expected. In these situations, nutritional geometry may be a useful method for examining the interactions between diet, nutrients, and liver health. The various dimensions and interactions between nutritional problems and NAFLD can be understood using models. Algorithms established by AI to build a customized diet for patients would be another significant contribution. But for a few broad dietary recommendations, the notion that there is no one-size-fits-all diet is gaining traction. Patients would most likely carry sensors that record details about what they eat in the coming years. This data would be combined with other data (physical exercise, tension, sleep, microbiota, biochemical constants, prescriptions, and genome) to include tailored dietary advice and nutritional counseling to avoid and manage NAFLD.

NAFLD (nonalcoholic fatty liver disease) is a widespread and possibly fatal type of chronic liver disease that affects people who do not drink alcohol. A low-calorie and low-fat diet are currently recommended for all Americans, particularly those with NAFLD. However, little is understood regarding the effects of diet quality on NAFLD patients' liver histopathology. The researchers decided to see whether average calorie consumption and diet structure were related to NAFLD histopathology's seriousness. From January 2001 to February 2002, seventy-four morbidly obese patients presented for bariatric surgery were retrospectively examined. Both patients received a preoperative nutritional assessment using a structured 24-

hour food recall, in addition to a regular surgical and psychiatric evaluation. Food consumption was calculated in terms of total calories and macronutrients, and the findings were linked to liver histopathology derived from normal surgery biopsies. The occurrence of inflammation or fibrosis and the magnitude of steatosis were measured separately using chi-square with categorical variables as well as ANOVA for continuous variables. In addition, for each histological result, we ran several logistic regression tests. There were no significant links between overall caloric intake and protein intake steatosis, fibrosis, or inflammation in the study. On the other hand, higher CHO consumption was linked to a significantly higher risk of inflammation, whereas higher fat intake was linked to a significantly lower risk of inflammation. Finally, current dietary guidelines can exacerbate the histopathology of NAFLD.